KT-386-799

RT84.5

000883

0176

QUEEN ELIZABETH COLLEGE OF NURSING

LIBRARY
SERVICE

CHANGING
NURSING
PRACTICE

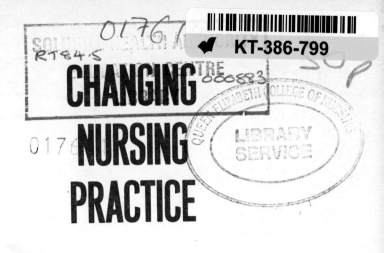

PLEASE BE ADVISED THAT THIS BOOK IS
AN OLD EDITION, NO LONGER REQUIRED BY
THE LIBRARY.

THEREFORE THE INFORMATION MAY BE
OUT OF DATE.

WITHDRAWN
FROM STOCK

60984 81800

YTISOHT

CHANGING NURSING PRACTICE

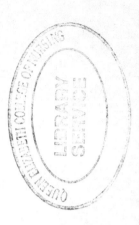

Stephen G. Wright
RGN, RCNT, Dip.N, RNT, DANS, MSc.

Consultant Nurse
Nursing Development Unit
Tameside General Hospital

With contributions by

Dirk Keyzer
RGN, MSc., PhD
Nursing Officer
Welsh Office

Lesley Surman
RGN, OND, RCNT
Nurse Teacher
Tameside General Hospital

Edward Arnold
A division of Hodder & Stoughton
LONDON   MELBOURNE   AUCKLAND

© 1989 Stephen C. Wright

First published in Great Britain 1989
Reprinted 1990, 1992

British Library Cataloguing in Publication Data

Wright, Stephen C.
    Changing nursing practice.
    1. Medicine. Nursing. Change. Role of nurses
    I. Title
    610.73'06'9

    ISBN 0-7131-4581-1

All rights reserved. No part of this publication may be reproduced
or transmitted in any form or by any means, electronically or
mechanically, including photocopying, recording or any
information storage or retrieval system, without either prior
permission in writing from the publisher or a licence permitting
restricted copying. In the United Kingdom such licences are issued
by the Copyright Licensing Agency: 90 Tottenham Court
Road, London W1P 9HE.

Whilst the advice and information in this book is believed to be true
and accurate at the date of going to press, neither the author nor the
publisher can accept any legal responsibility or liability for any
errors or omissions that may be made.

Typeset in 10/11 pt Palatino by Colset Private Limited, Singapore
Printed and bound in Great Britain for Edward Arnold,
a division of Hodder and Stoughton Limited, Mill Road,
Dunton Green, Sevenoaks, Kent TN13 2YA by
Clays Ltd, St Ives plc.

'Float like a butterfly, sting like a bee!'

Acknowledgements

Case study by Purdy and Wright (1988), *If I Were a Rich Nurse*, reproduced by kind permission of *Nursing Times* where this article first appeared on 12 October 1988.

Extract from the song *Good Friends* by Joni Mitchell reproduced by kind permission of Warner Chappell Music Limited.

I would particularly like to offer my thanks to Mrs M. McDermott and Mrs I. Hill for secretarial and other support above and beyond the call of duty.

Contents

Author's note

The words patient, client or resident are used interchangeably to describe the recipient of care. The reader is asked to interpret whichever they feel most comfortable with.

The word 'clinical' is used in the general sense; referring to any area where nurses are working directly with patients, clients or residents, in hospital or community.

Preface

'Knowledge is power.'

Hobbes   *Leviathan*

Every nurse has wanted at some stage to change nursing – not just in the grander sphere of things – but at local level, on a particular ward or unit. I remember by bungled efforts of the past when I assumed that, because I felt I was right, everybody would agree with me, and because I was wildly enthusiastic, everyone else would feel the same way too!

Ignorance is not bliss, it leaves you vulnerable, a pawn in the struggle for power and control which can occur when haphazard change, however well-intentioned, occurs.

The light began to dawn when I was fortunate enough to attend a course in which change theory and its application was covered in depth. Then it became clear that the skills needed to change things are as complex as any other – regardless of the level you are working at. I was able to take this knowledge forward and use it in my practice, in just the same way as I was familiar and skilled with the use of a blanket or a bedpan.

All three contributors to this book have gone through this experience. Becoming an effective change agent requires many complex skills to be developed – some nurses get there after many years of (often painful) experience. However, the path is both shorter and straighter if we have early access to the information we need. This book seeks to help in that respect, for it was the experience of all three contributors that, having learned the intricacies of change, there was a feeling that 'if only I had known that before'. Change theory, and how to apply it to nursing practice, is therefore the subject of this book. Knowing what to change is good, knowing how to change is better.

Tameside, 1989

Stephen G. Wright

For Ian

Introduction

Sometimes change comes at you
Like a broadside accident,
There is chaos to the order,
Random things, you can't prevent.
There could be trouble around the corner,
There could be beauty down the street.'

Joni Mitchell   *Good Friends*

If you have attended a meeting of nurses recently, then the chances are that the subject of 'change' has raised its head. It is hard indeed to pick up a paper, book or journal, or to switch on a television or radio, without finding the notion that 'things are changing' not just in nursing, but in the wider world around us.

Toffler (1973) writes of 'the roaring current of change, a current so powerful today that it overturns institutions, shifts our values and shrivels our roots. Change is the process by which the future invades our lives, and it is important to look at it, not merely from the grand perspectives of history, but also from the vantage point of the living, breathing individuals who experience it'.

This book seeks to address itself to the last point made by Toffler, for the three contributors have all functioned as change agents at clinical level; and much of what we write is based upon our own rich experiences. We wish to share these with you, because all nurses are caught up in change. We cannot avoid it. Like a lumbering beast entering a neat and well-protected garden, change threatens to enter all our professional lives. If we do not learn to master this beast, to ride it, and to steer it in the direction that *we* choose, then we can expect to be trampled beneath its hooves, ignored and trodden down.

So often in the past, this has happened to nurses. Powerless, apolitical and disorganised, we are swept along with change, able only to react and not control. Change is not only inevitable, it is accelerating, and nurses will face more and more of it in years to come.

In learning how to manage change, nurses can become effective change agents, but this is merely the beginning. The process of change, when set in motion, rolls on into the future as the change agent creates the 'clinical laboratory' (Infante, 1980) where others learn to accept change as a normal part of the culture.

Producing a climate of this nature is not easy for nurses, and in many ways it runs counter to the traditional perception of a professional. The tendency for professions to be elitist, controlling their members and their clients, is alien to the process of change advocated in this book. The nurse change agent works as partner and companion with both colleagues and client turning 'the servant into the master through the use of expertise' (Wilkes, 1981). Indeed, it may be argued that one of the traditional hallmarks of professions is the use (or abuse) of their powers to resist change. There is little need for nursing to become a pillar of the establishment, there are more than enough of these. Rather, nursing must advocate a new form of professionalism. In the acquisition of knowledge, skill, expertise or influence – some of the components of power – nurses can use these qualities not for their own self aggrandisement or to control others, but to empower others to take control of their destinies for themselves.

Campbell (1984) has argued that such a course is immensely difficult for nurses, for it demands altruism: 'the professional gains knowledge to help, but that knowledge gives both detachment and power. It is a hard demand that the detachment should not be used for the protection of self, nor the power for the enhancement of self'. The use of such power demands not only a love of the self, but a love of others in order to give of that power to help. Such a form of 'moderated love', states Campbell, underpins the ability of the nurse to act as a change agent.

The call to nurses to take on the mantle of change agency is also a call to take both political and personal action. The two need not necessarily be separated, indeed the position of nurses is a challenge for them to combine or hybridise the two. Halmos (1978) tends to segregate the two as distinct and incompatible forms of change agency. The political change agent is seen as partisan and tending to deal with people as massed groups (e.g., by different class, occupation or role). The personalist is less judgemental and focuses on dealing with individuals. The politicalist is characterised as domineering, using others to achieve their ends in Machiavellian style. The personalist works less certainly and is non-manipulative (Campbell, 1984). Nurses have the opportunity to be hybrids of these seemingly opposing poles. On the one hand they may work with individual colleagues or clients to produce awareness and assistance in change; or they might work to produce innovation in a small local way on their own ward or unit. On the other hand, they can participate in wider political movements, both inside and outside their profession and the organisations in which they work.

Clinical nurses are in a position to merge the two trends, to become hybrid change agents at personal and political levels, generating change in all manner of circumstances.

This book is aimed at such nurses and those who support them, be it on wards, in nursing homes or in the community. How often are we called upon to change things. Implement the process! Use a model! Change to primary nursing! These and dozens of other issues face clinical nurses today. It is relatively easy to attend a meeting or a conference and to learn *what* a new idea is all about. A quick lecture can soon fill us with the facts on a particular subject. The problem often arises when we try to put it into action. We can feel shocked and disillusioned when what we perceive to be a perfectly sensible idea is greeted with disbelief, resistance and even hostility from colleagues!

It is not surprising that nurses can find it difficult to be creative or to take on board new ideas. Surrounded by multitudes of pressures of work, and with your nose to the wheel and elbow to the grindstone, it is very difficult to look up and have a vision of new horizons! In addition, many nurses have not experienced progressive approaches which encourage them to learn to develop ideas and to put them into action.

Yet, as Toffler says, 'We are all in the business of change' and, if we are to manage that business well, we need to learn and practice its skills. Knowing what change is and how to take control of it can be learned, just like we can learn how to take a temperature correctly or give pills safely.

However, the opportunities to learn the skills of managing change are still relatively rare in nursing, unless we get there ourselves by dint of our own experience and intuition. Perhaps it is no accident that nurses are rarely taught to master change. The status quo of the social order, both inside and outside nursing, might feel a little uncomfortable at the prospect! For example, just imagine what a force for change the 500 000 nurses in the UK would represent! What would be the effects, not only on the health system, but also in society at large, if this army of skilled, assertive and aware change experts was unleashed upon them?

However, nurses must be skilful change agents for two principal reasons. Firstly, because nursing has the potential to contribute to the health and wellbeing of individuals and society as a whole. If we believe what we do is for the good of others, then we must ensure that we can better control what we do so that the recipient of our services, the patient or client, gets the best deal from us. Not everyone in health care always has the best interests of the patient at heart. As Machiavelli (1961) succinctly noted, 'the fact is that a man who wants to act virtuously in every way, necessarily comes to grief among so many who are not virtuous'. Changing and organising the health care system is like a giant game with a multitude of players. Playing the game while ignorant of its rules is doomed to failure. When nurses fail, they fail their patients too. Secondly, change produces stress for us as individuals. It is even more stressful if we feel that everything around us is beyond our control. We might resent the change because if frightens us or because we do not understand, but sooner or later change gets forced upon us for good or ill. Not all change makes things better! So we must be able to understand the nature of change, not only so that we are better able to determine its course, but also that we can protect ourselves. Many nurses are damaged humans as a result of change forced upon them, leaving them able only to react and resent.

Knowledge is power, and knowledge of change helps to give nurses the power over change. Thus armed we are not left merely to react, but may indeed be proactive in determining the course that nursing takes. Doing this, we serve not only the interests of ourselves but the interests of those we exist to help.

References

Campbell, A. V. (1984). *Moderated Love: A Theology of Professional Care.* Society for Promoting Christian Knowledge, London.

Halmos, P. (1978). *The Personal and the Political: Social Work and Political Action.* Century Hutchinson, London.

Infante, M. (1980). *The Clinical Laboratory.* The C. V. Mosby Co., St Louis.

Machiavelli, N. (1961). *The Prince* (Trans. by George Bull). Penguin, Hardmondsworth.

Toffler, A. (1973). *Future Shock.* Pan Books, London.

Wilkes, R. (1981). *Social Work with Undervalued Groups.* Tavistock Publications, London.

1

Meeting the challenge: strategies for implementing change

'It should be borne in mind that there is nothing more difficult to handle, more doubtful of success, and more dangerous to carry through than initiating changes in a state's constitution. The innovator makes enemies of all those who prospered under the old order, and only lukewarm support is forthcoming from those who would prosper under the new.'

Machiavelli *The Prince*

Change and innovation: an introduction to change theory

Whenever nurses meet to discuss the organisation and delivery of care, the issue of change is sure to be high on the agenda. Examples of the current changes taking place are numerous and include the introduction of nursing models in practice and education (Keyzer, 1985; Wright, 1986), manpower planning (Welsh Office, 1985), and the recent reorganisation of the National Health Service to introduce general management. Furthermore, organisations such as the United Kingdom Central Council and National Boards for Nursing, Midwifery and Health Visiting spend a great deal of their time and money making policy decisions to encourage innovation and change in nursing (UKCC, 1986).

Whilst change and innovation are ever-present in nursing organisations, it often appears that their chance of survival is slim (Keyzer, 1985). Research studies have isolated a host of professional, organisational, political and economic reasons why change in nursing organisations appears to be more apparent than real (Stacey *et al.*, 1970; Davies, 1980; Keyzer, 1985; White, 1986).

The problem facing nurses is not the inevitability of change, but the way in which the who, why, where, when and how of the process can be planned to achieve maximum benefit for individuals, groups, and society as a whole. Many attempts to implement change in nursing fail because of the unstructured approach adopted by the innovators, the lack of understanding of the nature of the change and the effect of the outcomes on the participants, or the lack of provision of resources needed to achieve the desired outcomes (Stacey *et al.*, 1970; Towell and Harries, 1979; Keyzer, 1985).

The purpose of this chapter is to explore the strategies available to nurses seeking to implement change in practice, education and management. Reference will be made to research studies utilising these strategies, but the more in-depth examples of change in nursing will be left to the other chapters of this book. The need to select a strategy to guide practice will be stressed and deemed central to ensuring the success of the venture, to clarify the nurse's thoughts on the nature of the change and to make sure that the outcomes maintain or promote the dignity of human beings. Thus the moral and ethical aspects of change are acknowledged to be part of the problem-solving exercise of planned change.

Definition of terms

The term change can be defined as an attempt to alter or replace existing knowledge, skills, attitudes, norms and styles of individuals and groups. It is a discontinuity of the subjects' past behaviours and their perception of that discontinuity. Change in nursing practice, education and management begins with existing structures and processes the plan for revising them, proceeds to the actions to achieve the desired outcomes and the evaluation of the success in creating something new or different. The altered form embodies elements of the previous one (Hall, 1977; Beyers, 1984).

Innovation can be defined as the introduction of new ideas, methods or devices. It refers to the material technology and the idea justifying that technology. Innovativeness describes a set of attitudes and values that are open to change. Innovation takes place in social systems over a period of time. It requires open channels of communication which permit the diffusion of new knowledge throughout the organisation (Hall, 1977; Keyzer, 1985).

The introduction of planned change can be viewed from two points of view: from the subjects' new behaviour, and as an example of innovation in the organisation. The process of planned change, therefore, involves the gathering of information on the innovation and on the nature and functioning of the organisation and its members. Thus, innovation in nursing practice includes the nurse, the resources available, the concepts and philosophies underlying the model for practice, and the way in which care is organised and delivered in the hospital and community setting.

The planning of change is a process in which the nurse takes deliberate actions to achieve the desired outcomes with the minimal use of resources. It is a problem-solving exercise in which the need for change and what needs to be changed is identified. The nurse plans the actions to achieve the desired outcomes, implements the plan, and evaluates the success of the venture. Parallels can be drawn between the framework used for the nursing process and the change process.

Strategies for change: meeting the challenge

The accelerated pace of modern life and the changes taking place within the provision of health care services demands that nurses develop their expertise in the management of change. Central to the facilities of change is the selection of strategies that are likely to achieve the desired outcomes. Just as the nurses would select a framework for practice, or to design the curriculum, choosing a strategy for change helps to clarify the nurse's thoughts on the nature of the change, and to plan actions in a logical and orderly manner.

Chin and Benne (Bennis *et al.*, 1976), in their discussion on the development of change theory, define the process of selecting a strategy as the deliberate and conscious use and application of knowledge as a tool for modifying patterns and institutions of practice. It involves a clear understanding of the elements of the situation, restructuring the elements in the most advantageous way, and finding the best possible solution to the problem at hand. Thus, selecting a strategy for change requires the nurse to have problem-solving, decision-making and communication skills. As such, the selection of a strategy for, and the planning of, change is a legitimate part of the professional nurse's role.

Haffer (1986) supports the problem-solving approach to planned change and suggests that, once the need for change has been identified, the nurse must match the strategy to the person(s) involved in the change. Haffer argues that two important issues need to be considered in selecting the appropriate strategy and to facilitate change. These considerations are:

the strategy should focus on the appropriate change target;
the willingness and ability of the group to change.

Towell and Harries (1979), in their discussion on innovation in patient care, also identified the need to consider how change could be

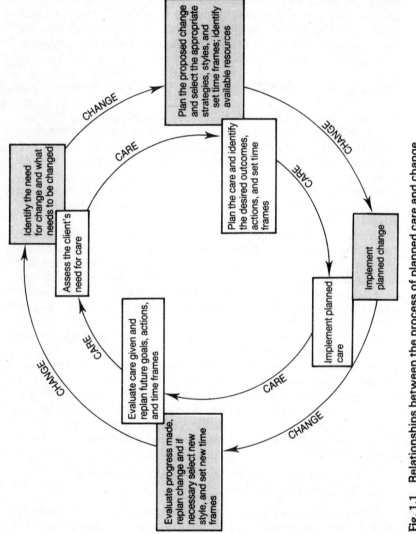

Fig. 1.1 Relationships between the process of planned care and change.

perceived by experienced nurses to be some form of criticism of past practices. In particular, they refer to the dominant features of large health care institutions which include a sense of isolation from the consumer of the service, a traditional rigidity and pattern of hierarchical dependence, a confusion in management and lack of collaboration between professionals, and a pessimistic climate in which awareness of resource constraints and memories of past failures inhibit individual initiatives. Similar conclusions were drawn by Keyzer (1985) who further identified the effect the distribution of power and control could have on the implementation of change. As nursing research develops our awareness of the factors which promote or inhibit change in practice, so also does it highlight the need to select a strategy, or strategies, which build upon the positive and overcome the negative elements.

Sugden (1984), Beyers (1984), Keyzer (1985) and Haffer (1986) all cite Bennis *et al.* (1976) and identify three predominant change strategies. These strategies are: rational–empirical; power–coercive; and normative–re-educative. Each of these strategies is based on different assumptions about what makes people change or alter their behaviour. Each strategy is viewed by Bennis *et al.* (1976) as having potentially different degrees of success. In discussing these three individual strategies, Haffer (1986) argued that the appropriateness of each strategy depended on the situation and the individuals whose knowledge, beliefs, attitudes, values or behaviour we seek to change. Thus, the nurse's expertise in identifying the source of the demand for, and the focus of, the change is critical to the selection of appropriate strategies. This in turn implies that change theory is an essential component in basic and post basic education programmes, and that students and trained staff need exposure to role models who value and support the implementation of change in practice.

The rational–empirical strategy

Chin and Benne (Bennis *et al.*, 1976, p. 24) call on a variety of strategies under the heading of rational–empirical. Underpinning this approach is the belief that all persons are guided by reason and that they will utilise some rational calculus of self-interest in determining needed changes of behaviour. This strategy is similar to Vinokur's model (1971) for decision-making in which it is suggested that, when faced with the possibility of choice involving risk, it is rational to select the outcomes offering the optimum value to the individual or group.

Examples of the rational–empirical strategy are the beliefs that the dissemination of research findings will change nursing practice, and that the distribution of leaflets outlining the spread of the disease AIDS will alter the population's sexual practices.

The power–coercive strategy

In the rational–empirical approach there is a basic assumption that knowledge is a major source and ingredient of power. Thus men and women of knowledge are power holders and the desirable change is achieved through the transfer of knowledge (power) to those lacking the specific knowledge in the education process (Bennis *et al.*, 1976; Bernstein, 1975; Keyzer, 1985). The power–coercive strategy as defined by Chin and Benne (Bennis *et al.*, 1976, p. 40) emphasises a different type of power. This power is based on the use of political and economic sanctions to achieve the desired outcome and, when necessary, the use of moral power. The common assumption underlying the power–coercive strategy is that persons with less power will always comply with the plans, directives and leadership of those with greater power. This strategy is one most commonly used and associated with the historical development of nursing organisations. Examples of this strategy are to be found in everyday practice, and range from the nurse manager's right to override the decisions made by clinical staff (Towell, 1975), to the government's directives for changing the structure of the National Health Service.

Both the rational–empirical and the power–coercive strategies can be viewed as 'top down' approaches to change. That is the need for change, the focus of the change, and the means of implementing and evaluating it, are identified by those in positions of power. The traditional attitudes of some doctors and nurses towards their patients, or teachers towards their students, provide examples of this practice. Thus, it is the doctor and the nurse who decide what the patient's needs are and how they are to be met. Similarly, it is the teacher who decides what the student needs to learn, how it will be learned, and what will constitute evidence of success or failure (Bernstein, 1975; Keyzer, 1985). Underlying these strategies is a belief in the inherent right of the power holders to exercise their power and the subject's uncritical acceptance of that right. There are many examples in both our social and professional lives to show how these strategies succeed and fail. The term 'noncompliance' is often used by nurses to describe patients who, for whatever reason, reject the nurse's perceptions of their needs for care.

Wright (1986) has argued that effective change in patient care is not only dependent on the selection of appropriate frameworks for practice, but also on the active involvement of the participants. Such a strategy is defined by Chin and Benne as normative–re-educative (Bennis *et al.*, 1976). This approach does not negate the inherent right of the power holders to define the need for change, nor to plan the actions to be taken. It seeks to reinforce these efforts to ensure the maximum benefits for all persons involved in the process.

The normative–re-educative approach

This strategy as defined by Chin and Benne (Bennis *et al.*, 1976, p. 31) rests upon assumptions about people that contrasts with those underlying the rational–empirical and power–coercive strategies. Chin and Benne argue that people need to be involved in all aspects of the change process and that their actions are directed by a normative culture which involves open channels of communication in social systems and agreed norms of behaviour. In this way, changes in practice are seen to involve not only the identification of a need for change by others and the provision of information supporting that need, but also the habits and values of individuals, and the structure, roles and relationships of, and within groups.

The normative–re-educative approach is a 'bottom up' type of strategy the success of which depends on the individual's or group's perceptions of the need for change and its relationship to daily practices. Towell and Harries (1979) support this 'bottom up' approach to change in nursing organisations and they provide examples of how the good ideas presented by the clinical staff can be supported to improve patient care. Similarly, Keyzer (1985), Pearson (1985) and Wright (1986), in their separate accounts of the introduction of nursing models in practice and education, have demonstrated the benefits of involving all levels of the nursing organisation in the change process. Thus, the normative–re-educative strategy is a means of bringing together the organisation's perceptions of the need for change (external needs for change) and the individual's, or group's, perception of the relationship of that change to the daily practice (internal needs for change).

Current examples of the application of the normative–re-educative strategy for change are the moves towards a more patient-centred and student-centred approach to care and education (UKCC, 1986). The active involvement of the patient in identifying his needs for care, selecting the actions to be taken to achieve the desired outcomes of the plan of care, and in evaluating the effectiveness of the care, is a normative–re-educative process of nursing (Pearson, 1985; Keyzer, 1985; Wright, 1986). Similarly, the devolved examination system adopted by the Welsh National Board of Nursing, Midwifery and Health Visiting affords the student greater control over the content of the learning programme and the assessment of the success achieved. The use of project work as part of the 'final' examination by the training institutions in Wales has demonstrated how the external needs of the organisation and the internal needs of the student can be met in innovative assessment strategies.

Selecting a strategy: some questions to be asked and answered

The three strategies for change are:

rational–empirical
power–coercive
normative–re-educative

Of these, the normative–re-educative approach appears to be the one most likely to achieve real change in nursing practice. It may be necessary, however, to utilise a combination of all three strategies to achieve the desired outcome. In which case, it is important to identify which strategy has been selected to achieve the various sub-goals of the proposed change (see Fig. 1.2).

To enable the nurse to select the appropriate strategy, a number of questions need to be asked and answered. The following questions should help the nurse to clarify the various components of the change process and to focus attention on the specifics.

Identifying the need for change and what needs to be changed

1 *What is it that you wish to change?*

   Is it a behaviour, an attitude, a skill associated with the introduction of new technology, the patient's health care practices, the student's knowledge base? A combination of all these factors?

2 *Why do you want to implement the change?*

   Is it because you have been asked to implement it by others (external source), or that you yourself have identified a need for change (internal source)? Is it that both you and your colleagues (group) have perceived a need for change? Is the change being enforced by senior members of the organisation (power–coercive), by the evidence found in research reports (rational–empirical), or is it being implemented because the group themselves have initiated the actions (normative–re-educative)?

Planning and implementing the proposed change

3 *How are you going to implement the change?*

   Are you simply going to issue an order (power–coercive)? Are you going to circulate information (rational–empirical)? Are you going to discuss the need for change with the subjects, listen to their opinions, involve them in all aspects of the process and provide supportive education programmes (normative–re-educative)?

4   *Where is the change to be implemented?*

Will the change be implemented in the classroom, the ward, the patient's home, the library? A combination of these sites?

5   *When will the change be implemented?*

Do you expect the subjects to implement the change in their own time or within their working hours? Are you going to set time frames within which the subsections and the whole change are to be achieved?

6   *Which resources will be needed to implement the change?*

Have you estimated the nature and quantity of resources needed to achieve the desired change? Will it require material, financial, manpower and educational inputs? If so, how much will it cost? Where are these resources coming from? Have you built in manpower resources to release staff from the clinical areas to attend the education programmes, or to reflect on the progress made? Who is going to supply the needed resources: the organisation, or some external agency in the form of a research grant?

7   *Who is going to implement the change?*

Are you going to implement the change yourself? Are you asking others to change their practice, learning and/or teaching strategies, or managerial styles? Will the change involve a group of clinical nurses, teachers and managers? Does the change involve other health care workers and, if so, have their needs been taken into account? Does the change involve the patient and his relatives and, if so, have their beliefs, values, norms and styles been taken into account?

Evaluating the change and replanning the next phase of the process

8   *What effect will the change have on the role of the nurse?*

In planning the proposed change have you defined the desired outcomes? Does the proposed change alter the role of the nurse and, if so, does it promote the role or diminish it? If the role is to be changed, have the tasks associated with the new role been identified and differentiated from those linked with the previous one? Does the new role alter the relationships held by the nurse *vis-a-vis* the patient, other nurse colleagues, the doctor and the manager?

9   *Which criteria are you going to use to evaluate the outcomes of the change?*

Are you going to use quantitative or qualitative evaluation methods to determine whether or not the desired outcomes have been achieved? Perhaps you will need to use both of these methodologies. Which tools are available to help you evaluate the change? Are there existing tools in the research studies supporting the change, or ones that have been developed by others attempting the same change? Will you have to develop new tools for the evaluation and, if so, is there local expertise to help you? Are you going to take the subjects' perceptions of the change achieved into account? Do you need complex computer services and programs to collate and analyse the evaluation data and, if so, are expertise and equipment readily available to you? Will you have to buy in expertise to help you analyse the evaluation data and, if so, where are the resources?

10   *How are you going to communicate the results of the change?*

Are you going to write a report of the implementation of change and the success achieved? If so, who is going to write the report? To whom may the results be communicated? Are you going to publish articles in the nursing journals? If so, who holds the copyright? Are you going to report back in a study day? If so, who is going to provide the resources for this study day? Are you going to involve the participants in the feedback to the group and others?

Once these questions have been answered, the selection of appropriate strategies leads to the clarification of the steps to be taken in putting the plan into action.

Putting the strategy into action

There is an increasing body of nursing knowledge (Pembrey, 1980; Keyzer, 1985; Wright, 1986) which identifies the leadership role of the ward sister in promoting and changing standards of care. Whilst the role of the ward sister embraces that of change agent, she cannot succeed without the full co-operation of her staff and other health care workers (Keyzer, 1985). In her daily practice, the ward sister needs to communicate, co-operate and negotiate with doctors, managers (nurse, unit and general managers), nurse colleagues and a host of other workers whose combined services are required to meet the goals of the organisation.

In formulating the plan of change, the nurse must consider how that change influences, and is influenced by, the services provided by colleagues. Beyers (1984) reinforces this need to acknowledge the recip-rocal relationships that exist within the health service and how change in any one part of the organisation affects the others. Thus, one of the prime functions of the nurse is to negotiate a mutual agreement for change within the nursing service and between the areas of the organisation.

In addition to selecting a strategy, or strategies, for change, the nurse must also select a framework which promotes the co-operation of colleagues and other work groups. Hersey and Blanchard (1982) offer a framework which helps the nurse to clarify thoughts about the rela-tionships between the amount of direction and support the change agent gives, and the degree of willingness and ability to change expressed by the participants. This model suggests four leadership styles the nurse can adopt to link the appropriate change strategy to the needs of the participants. These four styles (see Fig. 1.2) are:

telling
selling
participating
delegating

Telling
This style is a combination of the rational–empirical and power-coercive change strategies (see Fig. 1.2). An example is the decision taken by the statutory bodies to adopt nursing models and a problem-solving approach to care (GNC, 1977; UKCC, 1986). In this instance, the training institutions were provided with directives about a change in practice and education. Keyzer (1985) described how this policy decision was implemented and managed by one health authority. In this research study, the Nursing Policy Group adopted the patient-centred approach to care as official policy for all care areas. Seminars were then provided in which information was given to all nurse manag-ers and teachers. The nursing service then set up a Nursing Process Development Group to co-ordinate the implementation of this policy in the clinical areas. The service, therefore, exerted only a limited control over the adoption of this change.

This approach of 'telling' the members of the group is viewed by Haffer (1986) as being most suited to those persons of low ability and willingness to change, to take responsibility for independent action, or who feel insecure and unsure of their ability to change. Both Pearson (1985) and Keyzer (1985) provide evidence of the need to support individuals and groups who perceived a threat from the imple-mentation of the nursing process and the good effect information

Change strategy	Leadership style
Power–Coercive	*Telling* The change agent provides information, gives orders, directs change and defines the who, what, where, when and how of the change. Elements of rational–empirical strategy may be used.
Rational–Empirical	*Selling* The change agent provides information and attempts to convince the group of the need for change. Provides support for change, but is less directive than in the power–coercive approach. Elements of power–coercive and normative–re-educative strategies may be used.
Normative–Re-educative	*Participating* The change agent negotiates with the group in decision-making. Information and directions provided when asked for by the group.
	Delegating Self-directed change with minimal inputs from the change agent. The individual/group may adopt the change agent role.

Fig. 1.2 Relationships between change strategies and styles. After Bennis *et al.* (1976) and Hersey and Blanchard (1982).

giving had on the progress made. The need for supervision falls off as the individual or group gains confidence in their abilities to cope with and influence the desired change.

A further example of this style is to be found in any nurse training institution where nurse teachers adopt the traditional didactic approach to teaching nurse learners. Similarly, when students first set out to review the literature on a specific nursing subject, or attempt to initiate project work as part of their course, the nurse teacher may initially adopt a 'telling' style until the student gains the experience and confidence to control the contents of the assignment. The use of broad objectives for clinical placements may also be perceived as 'telling' both clinical staff and students about the learning opportunities available in the clinical areas. In this instance, the 'telling' styles provide the safety of a framework within which the student can explore the learning opportunities available without taking on responsibilities which belong to the teacher.

Selling
This style may contain elements of the power–coercive strategy, but utilises a more rational–empirical approach to change (see Fig. 1.2). Keyzer (1985), Pearson (1985) and Wright (1986), in their separate approaches to implementing nursing models in practice and education, provide evidence of utilising this approach. Keyzer (1985), for example, described the use of seminars, study days and workshops to help disseminate information on, and develop nursing expertise in, problem identification, problem-solving and the implementation of the nursing process. In this study, the nurses attempting to change their mode of practice were invited to contribute to these learning programmes and were, therefore, active in 'selling' the benefits of the new approach to patient care to others.

The benefits of this 'selling' style in this study were: the dissemination of the innovation to other wards, units and departments; the creation of a nurse advisory service between the nurses caring for elderly people in the general and psychiatric hospital; the setting up of a self-help education group between the units implementing the change; and the clarification of the nurses' thoughts about the process of nursing and the changes they had achieved (Keyzer, 1985).

Thus, the 'selling' style can be of most benefit when the nurse is dealing with clients who are willing to change, seeking direction, and/or require information to clarify the reason for change.

In the beginning, the change agent may have to provide the direction and information required by the client. As with the 'telling' style, this need for support wanes as the client gains confidence and expertise.

Participating
This style is described in the normative–re-educative approach to change and is the strategy appropriate to the needs of individuals and groups who are motivated, willing, and able to change (see Fig. 1.2). Thus a supportive, non-directive style, which permits the participants

to control the change and, which values their inputs, has the greatest chance of success (Wright, 1986; Pearson, 1985; Keyzer, 1985). Keyzer further describes such a group in the case study of the implementation of the nursing process in a psychiatric rehabilitation unit. In this case study, the charge nurses provided strong leadership and were supported in the need for change by some, but not all, of the staff. Group norms and values were used by the leaders to initiate support groups for those members of staff who had the ability to change, but were unwilling to do so through a lack of motivation or confidence. The charge nurses, in their roles of change agents, negotiated with the group to make decisions and set goals for the proposed change. In this way new nursing records were created; experimental shift systems were initiated; new attitudes to and behaviour of staff towards the patients were developed. Minimal directives were given by the external change energizers (the Nursing Process Development Group) nor were they sought (Keyzer, 1985).

One of the contributing factors to the success achieved by this group was that it had identified the need for change and selected a nursing model and process before the 'telling' and 'selling' strategies of the Nursing Process Development Groups had been initiated. Thus, the 'participating' style is most likely to succeed once the group have identified a need for change and have perceived its relevance to their daily practice (Keyzer, 1985).

Delegating
This style is an extension of 'participating' and is most appropriate for individuals and groups who have achieved a self-directed approach to change (see Fig. 1.2). Indeed, a self-directed, independent learning strategy is a perfect example of the 'delegating' style. It is the one most commonly used for students engaged in research studies. In this strategy, the change agent provides the minimal amount of support and only does so when asked by the group. Normative–re-educative strategies have the greatest degree of success and support the initiatives and independent actions of the individual(s) involved.

Whilst Hersey and Blanchard (1982) and Haffer (1986) perceived these situational leadership styles to be independent strategies, they could be seen to be steps in a continuum. There may be, for example, occasions when the nurse initiates the change by 'telling' the client about it, then proceeds to 'selling' the plan of change, goes on to support the 'participation' of the client in implementing the plan, and ultimately 'delegating' it to the client. Thus, these styles can be part of a problem-solving approach to planned change in nursing practice, education and management. All of these strategies and styles were utilised by Keyzer (1985) in an attempt to assist clinical nurses in implementing the nursing process in care of the elderly (see Fig. 1.3).

Group's response to change	Change strategy
Clinical nurses and teachers feel insecure and threatened by change towards implementation of the nursing process.	*Telling* Power–coercive. Statutory Bodies' directives to schools of nursing and midwifery. Policy endorsed by Nursing Policy Group.
Group gains greater confidence but feels insecure because of lack of information.	*Selling* Rational–empirical. Nursing Process Development Group set up to disseminate information and to identify and forge links with pilot areas.
Group gains confidence, but still requires support and information.	*Participating* Rational–empirical and normative–re-educative. Teachers negotiate learning contracts with clinical nurses to support move towards implementation of the nursing process. Groups become involved in study days and seminars on implementing the nursing process.
Motivation grows as group gains confidence in own ability to change.	*Delegating* Normative–re-educative. Pilot areas develop a self-help education programme. Teachers' roles change within the group and assistance is offered only when asked. Group publish accounts of the changes achieved.

Fig. 1.3 Examples of change strategies adopted by the author and clinical nurses attempting to implement the nursing process in practice and education. After Keyzer (1985).

Summary

The implementation of planned change in nursing organisations is a complex process which can be influenced by the individual's or group's perception of the need for change and its relationship to the daily practice of nursing. Furthermore, nurses need to consider how changes in nursing practice can effect the work of other health care groups and how these groups can promote or inhibit the achievement of desired nursing goals.

To ensure the success of any change in nursing practice, education or management, the nurse must negotiate with other health care groups. She or he must be able to convince others of the benefits of change in attaining the goals set out in the organisation's strategic plans. The support for, and the collaboration of others is more likely to succeed if the nurse has a framework for practice, which clarifies thoughts on the nature of the change and provides a process to implement the change in a logical and practical manner.

There are three strategies available to the nurse planning change in practice, education and management. These strategies are:

rational–empirical
power–coercive
normative–re-educative

Each of these strategies may be used on its own, but it is more likely that a combination of all three will be needed to meet the needs of individuals and groups. Furthermore, the focus of the change and the individual's or group's willingness and ability to change may dictate that these strategies be combined with different leadership styles. These leadership styles are:

telling the individual(s) to change
selling the idea of change to individual(s)
participating in the change process
delegating the control over all aspects of the change to the individual(s)

Whilst these strategies and styles may be seen as independent approaches to change, a combination thereof leads to a continuum along which the individual(s) may be found at any point in the change process.

The success achieved in implementing planned change will be influenced by the following.

• The active involvement of all levels of nurse and those whose practice overlaps the role of the nurse.

- Open channels of communication which permit the diffusion of the innovation throughout the organisation.
- The involvement of managers in supplying the resources needed to achieve the desired outcomes.
- The involvement of the teaching staff in supportive education programmes throughout and after the period of change.
- The participants' perceptions of the need for change and its relationship to their daily practice of nursing.
- The negotiations of flexible agreements between the change agent and the participants, and between the nursing service and other health care workers whose practice will be affected by the change.
- The active involvement of the participants in all aspects of the process and in setting time frames for the implementation and evaluation of the proposed change.
- The setting of standards and selection of criteria for measuring the outcomes of the change. This includes the individual's or group's evaluation of the success achieved.

Throughout this chapter, reference has been made to three specific nursing texts (Keyzer, 1985; Pearson, 1985; Wright, 1986). These texts have been chosen because they describe and evaluate the conscious application of change theory to the implementation of nursing models in practice and education. Each of these writers selected participating styles (see Figs 1.2 and 1.3) to underpin normative–re-educative strategies for change.

In their separate texts Keyzer (1985), Pearson (1985) and Wright (1986) have shown that clinically based nurses can effect change in nursing practice. Each identifies the constraints imposed by low staff: patient ratios, lack of understanding by others of the nature of the change and the distribution of power and control in nursing organisations. These factors do inhibit the progress made, but an understanding of how these variables effect our practice enables us to select different strategies and styles to minimise their influence. In this way, they exemplify that there is nothing so practical as a good theory when it comes to meeting the challenge of change in nursing practice.

References

Bennis, W. G., Benne, K. D., Chin, R. and Corey K. E. (1976). *The Planning of Change*. Holt Rinehart and Winston, London.
Bernstein, B. (1975). *Class, Codes and Control, Volume 4, Theoretical Studies Towards a Sociology of Language*. Routledge and Kegan Paul, London.
Beyers, M. (1984). Getting on top of organisation change, Part 1 Process and development. *Journal of Nursing Administration*, 14 (11), 31. Getting on

top of organisation change, Part 2 Trends in nursing service. *Journal of Nursing Administration*, **14** (11), 32–7. Getting on top of organisation change, Part 3 The corporate nurse executive. *Journal of Nursing Administration*, **14** (12), 32–7.

Britton, L. (1984). Use of behavioural science concepts and processes to facilitate change: a team building program for nursing supervisors. *Australian Health Review*, **7** (3), 162–79.

Davies, C. (1980). *Rewriting Nursing History*. Croom Helm, London.

General Nursing Council for England and Wales. (1977) *GNC Education Policy*, Ref. 77/19/A, HMSO, London.

Haffer, A. (1986). Facilitating change. *Journal of Nursing Administration*. **16** (4), 18–22.

Hall, D. J. (1977). *Social Relations and Innovation*. Routledge and Kegan Paul, London.

Hegyvary, S. T. (1982). *The Change to Primary Nursing*. The C. V. Mosby Co., St Louis.

Hersey, P. and Blanchard, K. (1982). *Management of Organization Behaviour* 4th Ed. Prentice-Hall, Hemel Hempstead.

Hockey, L. (1981). *Current Issues in Nursing*. Churchill Livingstone, Edinburgh.

Hollingworth, S. (1985) *Preparation for Change*. Royal College of Nursing, London.

Keyzer, D. M. (1985). *Learning Contracts, The Trained Nurse and the Implementation of the Nursing Process: Comparative Case Studies in the Management of Knowledge and Change in Nursing Practice*, PhD Thesis, London University.

Keyzer, D. M. (1986). Using learning contracts to support change in nursing organisations. *Nurse Education Today*, **6**, 103–8.

Keyzer, D. M. (1987). Contracting for change. *In Managing Change in Nursing Education*. Learning materials design for the English National Board for Nursing, Midwifery and Health Visiting. Newport Pagnell, Buckinghamshire.

Lancaster, J. and Lancaster, W. (1982). *The Nurse as a Change Agent*. The C. V. Mosby Co., St Louis.

Pearson, A. (1985). *Introduction of New Norms in a Nursing Unit and an Analysis of the Process of Change.* PhD Thesis, London University.

Pembrey, S. (1980). *The Ward Sister: Key to Nursing*. Churchill Livingstone, Edinburgh.

Peterson, M. E. and Allen, D. G. (1986). Shared governance: a strategy for transforming organisations. *Journal of Nursing Administration*, **16** (1), 1–12.

Porter-Stubbs, L. J and Wodniak, C. L. (1984). Theory nursing. *Nursing Success Today*, **1** (4), 27–30, 38.

Report of the NHS Management Inquiry (1983). Chairman, Roy Griffiths. DA (83) 38, DHSS, London.

Salaman, G. and Thompson, K. (1973). *People and Organisations*. Longman for the Open University Press, London.

Stacey, M., Dearden, R., Pill, R. and Robinson, D. (1970). *Hospitals, Children and Their Families*. Routledge and Kegan Paul, London.

Sugden, J. (1984). The dynamics of change. *Senior Nurse*, 1 (13), 12–15.

Towell, D. (1975). *Understanding Psychiatric Nursing*. Royal College of Nursing, London.

Towell, D. and Harries, C. (1979). *Innovation In-Patient Care*. Croom Helm, London.

United Kingdom Central Council (1982). *Education and Training, Working Group 3, Consultation Paper 1*. UKCC, London.

United Kingdom Central Council (1986). *Project 2000: A New Preparation for Practice*. UKCC, London.

Vinokur, A. (1971). Review and theoretical analysis of the elements of group processes upon individual and group decisions involving risks. *Psychological Bulletin*, 76, 231–50.

Welsh Office (1985). *First Report of the All Wales Nurse Manpower Planning Committee*. (WHC 85/32).

White, R. (Ed.) (1986). *Political Issues in Nursing: Past, Present and Future Volume 1*. John Wiley and Sons, Chichester.

White, R. (Ed.) (1986). *Political Issues in Nursing: Past, Present and Future Volume 2*. John Wiley and Sons, Chichester.

Whittacker, A. F. (1984). Use of contract learning. *Nurse Education Today*, 4 (2), 36–40.

Wright, S. G. (1986). *Building and Using a Model of Nursing*, Edward Arnold, London.

2

Theory into practice: some examples of the application of change strategies

'It has long been an axiom of mine that the little things are infinitely the most important.'
Sir Arthur Conan Doyle   *A Case of Identity*

Clinically based nurses can and do effect changes in nursing, constantly and continuously, but frequently without realising or understanding how it happened.

Passing through a hospital, or any centre where caring, management or education is taking place, it is possible to catch snippets of conversation (without intentionally eavesdropping of course!) which make reference to the need, the doing of, or the already having made changes to, existing practices. These come from all levels of staff, in all avenues, that combine to make the organisation which enables the caring of, and the caring for, people to happen. Nurses make up the largest percentage of the workforce among the caring professions. It is therefore important that they become aware that not only is it healthy for them to be introduced and subjected to new ideas but that they also can generate and perpetuate new ideas for themselves. There are a vast range of constructive ways in which individuals can contribute and participate to produce change and gain the rewards of their achievements.

Mauksch and Miller (1981) identify that 'the status of the individual who suggests new ideas seems to have great bearing on the manner in which new ideas will be accepted'. Sadly this is still true to a great degree. However, changes are afoot, and there are occasions when evidence of this can be seen.

During the course of this chapter, the strategies already identified (rational–empirical, power–coercive and normative–re-educative) will be examined in relation to clinical practice. Positive and negative case studies will be given to illuminate the advantages and disadvantages in adopting a particular strategy, either knowingly or innocently. In some instances, a particular strategy adopted has some characteristics of others.

Whilst all case studies are hypothetical and bear no reference to any person or persons known, it is hoped that they present a realistic and recognisable situation. It may be questionable as to whether change is needed, or indeed whether knowledge is advantageous in achieving a smooth, comfortable passage through this delicate operation of achieving change. The answer is undoubtably yes. The past has presented many occasions when the senior management has issued a directive, the junior wanting to be helpful and obliging says, 'yes sir', then proceeds to moan, be aggravated and even obstructive because they lack the information, knowledge or involvement to make them feel a real part of the suggested change. Instead they become frustrated that they are puppets to be manipulated at will.

Middleton (1983) identifies that potential nurses are chosen for having 'several basic characteristics which are inherent within a personality; these are in general agreed to be reasonableness, honesty, decency, honour and integrity'. The United Kingdom Central Council (UKCC) is now, through the professional Code of Conduct (1984), expecting nurses to retain these qualities. We need to ensure for ourselves and our colleagues, that these qualities do not diminish with time.

Case study 1   The innocent

Harold was a thirty-five-year-old gentleman who was admitted to hospital with a diagnosis of hypertension, obesity and constipation. The treatment he required was relatively straightforward and mainly concerned with education and the introduction of a healthier diet. The difficulties presented required careful re-education and adjustment to his life style. While this may be easy to say, it is in fact extremely difficult and hard work for any individual to make this adjustment and then maintain it.

On admission Harold was seen by the doctor who told him, 'We will give you some medicine to sort out your constipation and bring your blood pressure down, but you need to lose at least four stone in weight, that means a diet, and you will have to stick to it'. Harold found this rather depressing; he'd been on diets before and had had little success. Now it sounded rather serious. The nurses on the whole were quite nice but they only said the same things as the doctor. Harold began to feel that pressure was being put on him from the people with power. Unfortunately Harold was none the wiser as to how he was going to go about losing this weight; his experience of dieting had led him to believe his life sustenance was to consist of salads!! On his third day of admission, Harold found himself talking to a first year nurse. She had not been in training long and didn't seem bossy or upset to his expressing his moans and groans. Harold decided to ask this junior nurse some of the questions to which he had had no answers and which were now beginning to bother him. The junior nurse didn't have all the answers, but she listened and seemed to empathise with the tremendous upheaval Harold felt was about to change his whole way of living.

Over the following few days the junior nurse brought leaflets, cookery books, and ideas to Harold. He began to realise that life was not over. There were foods he could eat, if cooked correctly, his social life wasn't over, he could still go out and have a drink. Taking up exercise didn't mean five laps of the park before going to work, and importantly he didn't have to go it alone; there were groups and clubs which he could join which would enable him to share his agony with others in the same boat.

The junior nurse helped Harold adjust and come to terms with the changes he had to make to his life style in order for him to enjoy good health and wellbeing. She had little knowledge of the strategy of change she was employing, but the inherent qualities and characteristics expected, and quite innocently employed by this nurse, enhanced and nurtured a trusting relationship and promoted self-help in Harold.

This nurse and all nurses have the qualities and abilities to enable them to be change agents. Status on its own should not automatically lead an individual to perceive themselves as a radical/revolutionary change agent. The change suggested may be perceived as small or large, but it should always be given fair consideration and not discredited, ignored or undermined no matter who has offered the idea.

What is important is that nurses are educated and trained in using their inherent talents constructively. They must be given the knowledge to enable them to go forward into the ever changing world of nursing with confidence.

Before change is initiated, the change agent is advised to plan the change realistically, critically analysing the reasons for the change, identifying expected goals and outcomes, and his/her own attitude and that of the target group. Approach is all-important in effecting change. A problem existing for the change agent within nursing is that the target groups focused upon generally cover one, two or three decades of age differences. The training and education of nurses has changed considerably over the years and the acquired perceptions, values, views, opinions and practices of these individuals can conflict with regard to the requirements of each to enable them to accept change or participate in change.

The behaviour of the change agent is vitally important to the success or failure of an innovation. Change agents who were, and still are, perceived by themselves and respectfully by others as extremely good, innovative, creative and stylish change agents, have been known to attribute to others the resistance encountered towards change, instead of recognising that it is in fact being triggered by themselves. It is a hard and sorry lesson to have to learn through practice, and, in fairness, change agents are human too. Where it may sometimes be difficult to see and admit that the contributing factor to resistance is produced by oneself, if this can be achieved, the human support of a peer, colleague and friend can help the pain to dissipate and the 'what to do' be worked out. The person who acts as a change agent needs to have a high level of self-awareness, not only of how they personally respond, but also how they affect others. The target group need to feel involved and responsible. If the change agent can achieve this, then change will be seen to occur more quickly and smoothly.

The change agent must be careful not to present a superior attitude. He/she may have been the person to identify the change needed, why it is needed, perceive the outcomes of achieving the change, and identifying how to do it, but he/she alone does not herald the success. A feeling of trust and competence needs to be instilled into the group. The change agent must demonstrate an appreciation and understanding of the limitations and capabilities of the individuals who are to change, be involved in, or implement the change. It is therefore very important that the need for change must bear identifiable relevance. The target group must be able to positively identify with the benefits it should promote. They not only need to know why it is being postulated but also the expected goals and outcomes. Unclear change programmes, without understanding the rational, and with no clarification of actual and possible goals, is one reason for resistance from the target group.

There are, of course, other reasons for the resistance and it is frequently encountered with any movement away from the status quo. Insecurity within individuals, fear of the unknown, competition for power or influence, and limited resources may also be contributory factors.

Individuals or groups strive to achieve their personal goals and, therefore, challenge proposed changes. The challenge is not always realistic or justified. It is presented not with the view to how it may help the proposed area concerned, but how it may contribute to the individual attaining their own goals, and thus more influence and power. It is not so long ago nurses believed once they had completed their training, passed their exams and were admitted to the register, that they were then complete products and had no more to learn. Any nurse still believing this is sadly under a misconception and should prepare for an uncomfortable journey through nursing. The UKCC (1984) state that nurses should 'take every reasonable opportunity to maintain and improve professional knowledge and competence'. Each has a professional duty and responsibility to keep up to date with the latest findings; research, professional practice and developments. Nurses cannot afford to live on a day-to-day basis, they must look forward and anticipate changes which are going to occur; computerisation for example. To not comply with the computer requirements for practising nurses is not only unfair to his/her colleagues but potentially detrimental to themselves. It has to be remembered, too, that there is an obligation by managers and teachers to enable the nurse to meet these requirements. Ignorance is not accepted as a reasonable excuse, nor indeed is omission of action.

A favoured and much used resistance tactic is based in the past experience reference. If that experience was pleasant, more eagerness will probably be found in attempts to achieve change.

Case study II

It was the custom within this particular unit for the senior sister/charge nurse to cook breakfast for the staff of his/her ward who were on duty on Christmas Day morning.

The sister on the ward, enjoying this ritual, produced the full cooked English breakfast one year which the staff thoroughly enjoyed.

The next year sister thought they could try something different, a traditional Cheshire breakfast perhaps. The staff would not even contemplate it, 'the breakfast you cooked for us last Christmas was smashing, we'll have the same again this year thanks'.

There was no reason to change, everyone was obviously happy with last year's arrangements, so they enjoyed the same again. If the original experience had been negative, the prevailing attitude towards a fresh approach might have been different.

Case study III

Several years ago, in the formative stages of moving away from the task allocation and towards total nursing care, the 'work books' came under close scrutiny. The outcome was to recommend their removal from practice.

Whilst Nurse Brown, a third year student, was not alone in her disapproval of this change, her past experience produced resistance to the change, and a resulting bad experience.

Since the removal of the 'work book', nurses took to writing copious notes on scraps of paper which they then kept in their pockets for reference. It was the practice of the night nursing officer to do 'a round' with the nurse when she visited the ward at night; name, age, religion, diagnosis of patients all had to be recited. Nurse Brown was so worried about being told off if she did not know all the information that it went down on a piece of paper and into her pocket, to be pulled out when 'the round' came.

Nurse Brown survived 'the round'; tired and relieved she went off duty at 8 a.m. Whilst walking through the hospital, she put her hand in her pocket to get a tissue. On pulling out the tissue she dropped her information-laden piece of paper. Unfortunately, it was found and read by relatives who had been called in to see a patient whose condition had deteriorated and who was referred to on the nurse's notes. The diagnosis of 'Ca Bronchus' was on the piece of paper, neither the relatives or the patient had been told. There resulted much upset and unrest. Nurse Brown was disciplined.

Some years later, Nurse Brown, then qualified, found herself working with a progressive and innovative sister, in an area where the nursing process had been introduced. Sister James proposed that the care plans should be kept at the end of each bed. There was no way Nurse Brown could bring herself to work this new practice, her past experience blinded her to any advantages it had, all she felt was acute stress and fear. She obstructed the change in any way she could, overtly and covertly. Eventually she left to move to another area.

The past experience, although not totally related, bore strong enough resemblances for Nurse Brown for her to view this with only a negative perspective. When faced with a negative response it is helpful to analyse the two situations, identify areas that will be different in approach, execution, and/or expectation, in an attempt to win the unconvinced over before either discarding the idea or proceeding with it.

Achieving change needs careful consideration from the onset; most importantly in the area of communication. Inadequate communication and support from the top level increases apathy and sponsors a lack of involvement amongst the nurses; interest is lost and co-operation diminishes. Whilst there must be agreement on the goals and probable and possible outcome, one must estimate if this is realistic when considering the requirements to achieve it.

If the time is insufficient, staff turnover is such that it promotes inconsistency and if finances are inadequate to accomplish the change with a degree of success, it is questionable if the change should be embarked upon. Change is threatening to those with the broadest of outlooks, let alone those who cannot see beyond the conclusion of the task in hand. Failure is demoralising and will make attempting innovation and change extremely hard to contemplate within this group again. It is, therefore, best to ensure that, as far as possible, the resources are there to fulfil the change successfully. Starting off with a small scale scheme can be helpful; a quickly achieved goal (and recognition of it) can do much to reinforce the morale of the staff for grander changes to come.

The final form of resistance is passive, which is often inactive and concealed. Inefficient, stubborn or sullen behaviour are all symptoms of passive resistance. It is thought to manifest itself as a result of suffering difficulty in controlling one's own work environment or in directing change for themselves (Cooper *et al.*, 1987). The change agent, having assessed his/her own attitudes and behaviour and that of the target group, then needs to go on to implement the change, using the most appropriate strategy. As described in the previous chapter, there are choices of strategy to be made.

Examples of different strategies in the clinical situation

Power–coercive (telling)
Change is mostly recognised as 'top-down' directives. We are 'told' what to do, 'when' to do it, and 'where' to do it. Unfortunately the 'why' and 'how' it must be done is often missing. The answers are important though in achieving success in change. Traditional 'top down' style management appears to be common in the NHS (Price Waterhouse, 1988) which inhibits the opportunity which nurses have to be creative change agents at clinical level.

Many policies and procedures are laid down by management in many settings, and are issued to clinical areas where the staff are expected to implement them without question. The presentation style of documented procedures has, over the last few years, seen a change. There is a definite, positive and well-needed move away from the directive approach of documentation towards principles as guidelines to practice. However, the procedure book 'bibles' exist in many places.

> *Case study IV*
>
> The aseptic technique procedure was written as a directive. 'The nurse must wash her hands and dry them before laying up her trolley. The nurse must prepare her trolley and the patient, wash her hands again and dry them on a sterile towel provided in the dressing pack prior to commencement of the aseptic technique.'
>
> In good faith, the most appropriate people were asked to write the policy and procedure, being members of a surgical ward. The

policy and procedure allowed for patients to be taken to a specific area for aseptic procedures to be conducted; sound practice and highly commendable. It did not, however, take into consideration, for example, the care of the elderly areas where frequently the treatment room was no bigger than a wardrobe, hence dressings would have to be carried out at the bedside. The problems which then arise from nurses adhering to 'rules' are quite dangerous. The nurse washes her hands thoroughly before commencement of the aseptic procedure, but then walks a distance of what may be 20 metres, dripping water all over the floor and picking up an abundance of airborne micro-organisms on her warm, wet, well-exposed hands and arms during the course of her journey, and then has to manipulate her way through the drawn bed curtaining just to dry her hands on a sterile towel.

Sadly, the disillusioned then believe their hands and arms to be sterile, and the potentially dangerous spots of water all over the floor are justifiable for the cause. This is not so; the nurse may have adhered to the written rule, but has not demonstrated an understanding of the principles of asepsis, nor demonstrated skill.

In more recent years, this procedure has been rewritten and presents more as guiding principles. 'The nurse must wash her hands thoroughly and dry them well before laying up her trolley. The nurse must prepare the working area of her trolley and prepare the patient. Then thoroughly wash and dry her hands again prior to commencement of the aseptic procedure.'

The subtle difference in the wording of the procedures does, in the second instance, allow for the practitioner to continue to work at a level where rules are adhered to, but also demonstrate skill mastery in all domains, and comply with professional requirements. While such policies may be set up to protect patients and ensure certain standards, they may be adhered to rigidly or rejected by staff who are not allowed or feel unable to use their initiative, or who resent an 'order' being imposed from elsewhere.

Case study V

Whilst visiting the wards of a rehabilitation unit around the lunch time period, a visiting manager was appalled to see the beds were still in disarray. The ward looked untidy as an outcome of this and the manager was most displeased. Two days later, a memo arrived for the wards of that unit stating that all beds on the wards must be made by 11 a.m.

The staff were upset and angry on receipt of this memo as they had been given no explanation of why this was so essential, and no opportunity to state their reasons for this not being assessed as a priority of morning duties. The memo served only to reinforce amongst the staff that belligerent bureaucracy was still alive and thriving. There was good reasoning for the practice of leaving beds unmade; it was part of the patients' therapy to make their own beds.

The memo was discussed at a staff meeting and the consensus of opinion remained that they would be failing in their responsibility to the patients and the execution of their treatment if they changed their organisation of priorities. Consequently, the majority of beds remained unmade until after 11 a.m. There was no positive outcomes from this power–coercive strategy, and no positive change occurred. It did, however, serve to strengthen negative attitudes towards management; trust, morale and the feeling of achievement from work well done were all diminished. Even putting honourable, constructive change proposals to this group of people was met with hesitation, wariness and degrees of resistance for some time after.

Rational–empirical (selling)

This approach assumes that people are going to view change in a positive manner and work constructively towards it if they are given the basic facts, and so long as there is some evidence that they will derive a degree of benefit from the change. As previously identified, the target groups in the caring field usually comprise members with differing age ranges. Basic facts which are sufficient and acceptable to one generation may well not be for others. Using this strategy, the change agent uses persuasion; attempts to sell the proposed change by offering inducements, incentives and rewards, or suggests that new knowledge provides a sound reason for change.

Griffiths (1983) made a study of the National Health Service; the result of which produced another massive reorganisation within management levels. One of the many outcomes from this was the transferring of responsibility for ward budget expenditure and control to the ward manager. This is an onerous responsibility for which the majority of ward managers were neither prepared, nor wished to take on.

Case study VI

Study afternoons were arranged for sisters to attend where their new budgetary responsibilities and assessment of requirements and expenditure would be explained to them. A lot of time was spent describing the important step and how it would benefit both patients and staff. The incentive was that each ward would receive a percentage of their expenditure savings to be used in whatever way the ward wished. Although this sounded quite attractive, actual figures were lacking (as at the end of the day was the money).

In this instance, not only were the new budget controllers not fully told the whole aim, nor given realistic goals and outcomes, but no one advised them how to go about achieving this without lowering standards. A great moan from many new budgeters was not so much the saving of money, most knew that money could be saved in some areas (although not in the quantities requested nor with the repetition year after year which had been specified), but where the time was to come from. What should they give up in order to meet these new responsibilities?

On the whole, two years later at least, few, if any, ward budget holders are any wiser; they remain bewildered, pressured and disheartened, and very tired! They also remain uncertain as to what their individual budgets are.

This is possibly an instance where little progress was likely to be made, and it is hardly surprising that the proposals were met with a multitude of resistance strategies.

The introduction of the nursing process and patient allocation is another example of change which met with animosity (Wright, 1986). Indeed, in some establishments its introduction was of a power-coercive style, which then progressed to the more used rational-empirical strategy to enable any degree of success to be attained. The target group for this change already had many converted members and others who were able to be sub-agents. It is, however, a good example of how long change can take. The English National Board estimated ten years for the change to be complete, yet there is still a long way to go before it can be said to be established and working to its full potential nationally. There are still individuals who are not convinced of the need for this change, but more have been 'sold' the idea and are enjoying the benefits it brings.

Case study VII

Sarah Walker, a qualified nurse for eight years and a sister of a busy medical ward, was, like many other sisters, given the paperwork and forms and told to introduce the nursing process on Monday morning of next week. She was by nature quite progressive and well-respected by her staff, but even Sarah had trouble with this change. She felt rather hurt and as though she was being told that, after all this time, she wasn't doing things right. All that paperwork, how on earth was anyone supposed to get it filled in, as well as getting everything else done? The most disappointing aspect was the lack of support from the managers who had told her to implement it. The other sisters felt very much the same, although some, like Sarah, felt that there were positive aspects to this change but didn't understand them fully enough to convince staff to put in the effort.

Sarah already had a place on the Diploma in Nursing course and hoped that the course would help her to perceive the benefits of the nursing process with more clarity. As the course progressed, Sarah did understand with more clarity and her enthusiasm fired afresh. She was able to help her staff and convince them of the need for this change. She found enjoyment in giving them the time and support, and ultimate pleasure for all in finding the morale of the staff and standard of care improving. It still took Sarah three years to establish the nursing process and patient allocation fully in her area, partly due to management making full use of Sarah's enthusiasm and sending her staff to be trained and educated (or converted) to the nursing process.

As Sarah's understanding grew, her style of change strategy gradually underwent adaptation. As this style of nursing became the norm for Sarah, so her change strategy became one of normative–re-educative.

Normative–re-educative

The previous chapter has suggested that this is the most effective strategy in influencing change in the long-term. The change agent encourages participation and delegates responsibility. In this strategy, the change agent may be an active or passive member of the group, giving information, advice and direction when it is required and asked for, but allowing the group to motivate and direct itself, with possibly decreasing involvement of the initial change agent as the competence and confidence of the group increases.

Nurses need to continually review their beliefs, values, opinions and practices, not only because of the demands of the nursing profession on its individual members, but also because of the demands of the public. This is easy to say in theory, but not always so easy to do in practice.

Case study VIII

Talking to a retired nursing sister about changes which had occurred in nursing during her practice, she told of the time when Hugh Jolly, an eminent paediatrician, joined the hospital she was working at as a new consultant.

'I remember when Hugh Jolly joined us, he wasn't so much a breath of fresh air as a gust of wind. Of course, it was a long time ago, he was young then. Suddenly the doors were always open to the parents, radios were on, the kids were allowed to play and make a noise, I think they even got a fish tank – with fish in it.' A quiet smile came to her face as she went on to say, 'matron had a blue fit . . . but we thought it was wonderful!'.

Change always brings new experiences and, as more details are known of how we may go about achieving change, then it is hoped that the experience it gives will be of a positive nature. It is quite exhausting for those with established practices to have to embark on tearing them apart. The approach is all-important in promoting willingness and motivation in members of the target group (the change agents' attitude was discussed earlier).

This strategy, it has been suggested, is best used when approaching individuals who are motivated, willing and able to change. Many individuals can, however, be re-educated to this state.

Case study IX

Sister Harrison took the senior sister's post on a long stay and, supposedly, care of the elderly ward. Routines were well-established and the days ticked by with little stimulus or adventure. Being sited in a hospital, the ward had always followed the visiting hours of 2.00–3.00 in the afternoons and 7.00–8.00 at night. The rigidity of these visiting times had always bewildered Sister Harrison. If she could establish open visiting, maybe the patients would get more visitors and be awake when they came, they could be more involved (lots of advantages in that) and, hopefully, some life and fun would return to the ward.

Management had no objections to whatever visiting hours Sister Harrison adopted. The ward was in the old workhouse and so far removed from the main hospital that the hours did not really matter.

To Sister Harrison's amazement, the staff were appalled at the idea. 'Visitors get in the way, they want to be involved with their relatives and they ask a lot of questions.' 'At least during visiting hours we can get out of the way.' 'We can't get things done when visitors are around, apart from that, what if they come when the ward is untidy?' These were some of the retorts she received.

These responses served only to reinforce her niggling suspicion that the ward functioned with not much active thinking on the part of the staff. The thought of a sudden invasion of relatives, who were apparently to arrive in droves and stay for 24 hours, seemed to threaten them terribly.

Talking about the positive aspect of open visiting achieved nothing, or so she thought. While Sister Harrison was pondering how she should proceed, for achieving this small thing for her patients she was determined to do, she was approached by two of her staff, a staff nurse and an enrolled nurse, who, having had a few days to think about and consider what Sister had said, wanted to express their agreement and support. This gave Sister the starting point she needed. Negotiation with other members of the staff at a general ward meeting led to agreement in extending the visiting hours; 10.00–11.30 a.m., 2.00–4.30 p.m. and 7.00–8.00 p.m. Considering the animosity with which the suggestion had originally been met, Sister Harrison was delighted. The progress was not as slow as had been expected and the benefits of extended visiting hours were reinforced. The patients were certainly happier and the visitors appeared more friendly. The staff soon adjusted to the visitors' presence and 'visiting hours' gradually dissolved and open visiting became the accepted norm.

Summary

Whilst being 'told' what to do can be a comfortable way of functioning for many people, the effectiveness of any particular task carried out is of better quality when the individual concerned knows why it should be done in a given way. Effecting change is not so different. As the target groups can be of such diverse characters, the approach, level and strategy adopted must be compatible with their abilities. If resources of any kind are required, the change agent and managers have a responsibility to ensure they are available.

Support is essential, especially in the early stages. Individuals have a vested interest in maintaining the status quo in terms of their own ego and power. Change creates uncertainty and anxiety. It questions longstanding and established practices which can undermine the individual's self-esteem. The type of support needed varies for each individual during the course of implementing change. The commitment of the managers and change agents is essential, but support can be gained from the peer group(s) and recipient group(s) as well.

A positive attitude towards achievement of the goal of those involved is essential. Involvement as early as possible is beneficial. In this way, the individuals become interested, their commitment is gained, and the rewards reaped, not just in productivity, but also in the individual's self-esteem.

To return to an earlier example, in many establishments the background work for the introduction of the Nursing Process was completed before the target group was approached. The forms were designed, the style and presentation prepared without consultation and involvement of the target group. The instruction to change to this new type of nursing was met with much animosity. Involvement of the target group at the planning stage could have alleviated many problems and promoted an earlier attainment of success. The strategy of change adopted in the early stages of any innovation may be different to the style in which it is completed.

The needs and requirements of the target group may change and, with this possible occurrence in mind, change agents should continually be observing, assessing and evaluating their strategy. An innovation such as the Nursing Process, which started with power–coercive change strategy, has, through time in many establishments, been continued using an rational–empirical strategy. Today, in most instances, the emphasis has shifted to a normative–re-educative approach.

That change is inevitable is a fact that nurses must accept. The better equipped they are to be involved in its execution, the better it must be for nursing.

References

Cherniss, C. (1981). *Staff Burnout: Job Stress in the Human Services*. Sage, London.

Cooper, C., Cooper, R. and Eater, L. (1987). *Living with Stress*. Penguin, Harmondsworth.

Griffiths, R. (1983). *Management Structure of the National Health Service*. Report to the Secretary of State.

Harward, D. (1979). *Power: Its Nature, Its Use and Its Limits*. Schenkman, Boston.

Lazarus, M. and Lannier, R. (1978). Stress related transactions between person and environment. *In* Dervin. L. A. and Lewis, M. (Eds), *Perspectives in International Psychology*. Plenum, New York.

Mauksch, I. G. and Miller, M. H. (1981). *Implementing Change in Nursing*. The C. V. Mosby Co., St Louis.

Middleton, D. (1983). *Nursing I*. Blackwell Scientific Publications, Oxford.

Price Waterhouse (1988). *Recruitment and Retention of Nurses*. Price Waterhouse, London.

Wright, S. G. (1986). *Building and Using a Model of Nursing*. Edward Arnold, London.

3

The nurse as a change agent

'Prometheus by his free will undertook and carried out responsibly his plan, though he knew very well the consequences of his action. He had other alternatives, but he chose the nobler one and committed himself to his decision, which was to help men do better by making them masters of their minds.'

Vassilike Lenara *Heroism as a Nursing Value*

Why should nurses change (either themselves or the world around them) at all? It seems that the pressures for change are both external and internal. On the one hand, there are the changing needs of society and the political and economic forces which impinge on nursing. Pressure for change may come from governments, or professional organisations. This may be reinforced when those who make use of nursing, the patients or clients, as well as the potential consumers, find that all is not well with nursing. On the other hand, nurses themselves may come to an awareness that they could not only do things differently, but better.

Not all change is necessarily a change for the better, but nurses are in a weak position to judge this unless they are aware of who they are and what they do, and are able to articulate it to others. Achieving such a status may take many years, on the long road from novice to expert, as described by Benner (1984), but nurses at least seem to be becoming connoisseurs of nursing, if the explosion of literature about nursing by nurses in the last ten years is anything to go by.

It is perhaps the failings in nursing practice which give most genuine cause for concern. These might be identified by nurses themselves or those who make use of their services. The opportunity for the latter to express their views should increase with the growing acceptance of quality assurance methods which involve patients and clients. The test of nursing's success therefore seems to come from three directions, as shown in Fig. 3.1.

When nurses are required to change their practice, it takes expert nurses to judge whether the change is in the best interests of their

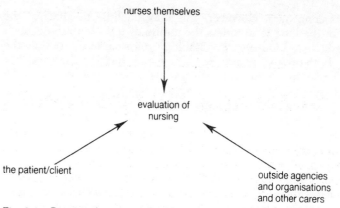

Fig. 3.1 Perspectives on nursing.

patients. Unfortunately, many nurses still lack the knowledge and skills to be able to do this and they find themselves unable to resist negative changes when they are imposed upon them.

The institutional, hospital based emphasis on nursing this century has produced many deep-seated problems for nursing. Historically, much of the training of nurses has taken place in hospitals (Beyers and Philips, 1971). The dangers of the institutionalised approach to care by the carers, which develops in the 'total institution' (Goffman, 1961), should not be underestimated. Nurses, like any other discipline, can develop an institutionalised attitude to work, just as the patient himself can become institutionalised in the hands of the carers. Once socialised into this attitude, the nurse will act it out. In an effort to bring order and control to the working day, the nurse can inflict upon the patient a degree of order and control which denies the patient even the most basic of human rights, dignities and freedoms.

Martin (1984) explored many of the failings in such a setting, including:

negative values related to nursing and patients
lack of leadership
lack of development/knowledge of the staff
lack of resources
lack of involvement of staff and patients in the decision making
    process
poor facilities, buildings, etc.

Unfortunately, when such problem hospitals have hit the headlines, there has been a tendency to search for scapegoats and to punish the 'evil' staff concerned. However, this may do little to alleviate the problem in the long term unless the nature of the institution is itself challenged. 'Individual psychopathology may have a part, but the issues are both broader and deeper. They are broader in the sense that much turns on the attitudes of society to its weakest members, and the resources assigned to their care; they are deeper in that what may occur is a perversion both of individual motives and of social institutions' (Martin, 1984).

The effects of the institutional approach are not confined to hospitals. Nurses and other carers at work in the community can develop and display similar attitudes – witness the recent report into the Nye Bevan Lodge (Gibbs *et al.*, 1987), the Yorkshire Television investigative documentary (YTV, 1986) or the growing evidence of abuse of those being cared for in their own or their relatives' homes (MacDonald and Rich, 1983).

Abuse is not always so dramatic or demonstrable, often it is subtle, hidden and carried out in the most well-intentioned manner. The tendency of the nurse or other carer, lacking knowledge, time or resources, is to take control of the patient's life. 'Let me do that for you, it will be quicker' – reinforcing dependence, and helping the carer, at least in the short term to 'get through the work' (Clarke, 1978) more quickly.

While the worst excesses of nursing failings (at least those which are reported) are relatively rare, there is no room for complacency. There is a need to be a constant watchdog over the service that is provided, to be aware of what needs changing and how best to go about it; whether it involves the nurse changing herself, or confronting the organisation with its own errors and inadequacies.

Who are the change agents?

Change agents may be people who are brought in from an outside organisation to change things, e.g., a consultant from a managerial company brought in to advise on the reorganising of a department. Alternatively, the change agent may be someone who works within the organisation who provides the expertise to make changes. Of course, not everyone wants or is able to change things. Nursing might be seen as being particularly disadvantaged in this theme, not only because we have yet to mature as a profession which can clearly articulate what it is, but also because it is a female dominated organisation, which has not traditionally been taught the skills of leadership. 'It is all very well being urged to provide leadership, but difficult in practice, especially as so few of us have been adequately prepared for

such a role. Nursing particularly suffers from the fact that qu
such as leadership are not seen as socially or culturally appropriat
the women who comprise over 90% of its workforce' (Salvage, 19

What does seem clear is that the potential to be a change agent lies,
to a greater extent, in every nurse. Each nurse may approach change in
a different way and with varying degrees of enthusiasm.

Rogers (1962) suggests that any given body of workers will vary in
their responses to the challenge or threat of change. The leaders in
change innovation come from a small minority, with their followers
gradually adopting the new ideas over time until only a few change
resistant or 'laggards' remain.

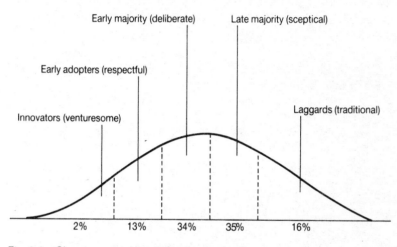

Fig. 3.2 Change – the responses by the staff.

The change resisters can produce disharmony in the setting, hold up
progress, or form 'cliques' to support one another. What is taking place
in the change setting, as it takes on new values and new directions,
may leave the resisters feeling isolated. Ultimately, if the change
becomes adopted permanently, they may vote with their feet – by
leaving. Thus, in some settings where change is taking place, the
organisation has to be prepared that some staff may leave when they
finally feel they cannot be a part of the team.

There is an obligation on the part of the change agents and those
who support them to involve the whole team in the change process and
endeavour to bring even the most resistant of the laggards along with
them – through education, support, rewards, and so on. Ultimately,
however, some will go, but this should not be a major problem as
those who replace them, if aware of the setting to which they are

going, are likely to already accept the values of the organisation which they have chosen to work in.

Ottaway (1980) analysed the different types of change agents and develops Rogers' (1962) ideas further:

Change generators
a)   Prototypic – the 'hero' type, changing hearts and minds with passion, enthusiasm and charisma.
b)   Demonstrative – of which there are three 'subspecies'
   i)   'barricade' demonstrators – the demonstrators at barricades or on the streets, often at the front line of conflict
   ii) 'patron' demonstrators – benefactors of the change process, e.g., giving money or appearing at meetings to offer support
   iii) 'defender' demonstrators – representatives of those who will benefit from the change, e.g., an elderly person speaking up at a public meeting to support changes in a local hospital.

Change implementors – once a need for change is recognised they are brought in to implement it. They may be:
a)   External change implementors – invited in, e.g., on a 'free-lance' basis to help the staff.
b)   External/internal change implementors – e.g., a nurse teacher working on one site, but visiting others to assist with developing new ideas.
c)   Internal change implementors – work with their own peers and colleagues within the organisation to change things.

Change adopters – fall into three types:
a)   The prototypic change adaptor – their task is to be the first adopters of the change in the organisation.
b)   Organisation maintenance change adopters – they can be very resistant, but may adopt the change in order to preserve as much of the rest of the system as possible.
c)   Product (service) users change adopters – in the service a product accepted by the user, e.g., the patient.

Ottoway's interesting taxonomy indicates that the change generators are often mistrusted in the organisation, that they like to effect change quickly and move on, and that they have very well thought out values. Change implementors work on the 'felt need theory', i.e., helping people to change because they have come to feel that they want to. They are often seen as more trustworthy, working with colleagues to sell their ideas.

The change adopters form the mass of change agents. Their task in the process is to take up the change, but they are often unaware of their role in the process. This reaches down through all grades of staff and ultimately to the consumer; the patient or client. When this succeeds, patient and staff satisfaction are in harmony, when it fails, there can be problems.

> *Example*
> The staff on a ward gradually adopt a 'progressive' approach to care, removing restraints on elderly patients. The patient's relatives complain that the staff 'don't care' any more because they do not appear concerned with safety. The change, the need for it, or the philosophy behind it, has not seen 'sold' to the relatives and the patient.

Rogers' and Ottoway's models may seem rather complex, but they do offer an opportunity for the nurse who would be a change agent to assess.

• Where do I fit in among these types? Am I a particular one, or do I have qualities akin to many. If so, how will my colleagues perceive and react to me?
• Where do all my colleagues fit into these models? Who will support and who resist? What strategies can I use to deal with these?

The shifting sand effect
Imposing change in any setting can be likened to taking a walk along a beach when the tide has just retreated. The wet sand is inviting, ripe for having new impressions made upon it. Thus some nurses try to change things. Entering upon virgin territory, they stamp their mark upon the staff and the way they work. The footprints are deep and obvious, like those on the wet sand. But, as the innovator walks on, the footprints gradually fill in, the sand returns to what it was before, and nothing has changed. Imposing change in any setting may be successful on the short term but, ultimately, it fails.

Scheff (1967) described the concept of 'front line organisations' – the ability of groups of workers to ignore or manipulate the orders that the boss has given. Thus, the innovator may believe that change has occurred because they ordered it but the reality is that, in their absence (when they leave, or simply go 'off duty'), the system reverts to what it was before. How many ward sisters have implemented a change on the ward and gone off for the weekend suspecting that, as soon as their backs are turned, the staff are 'up to their old tricks again'?

Ownership
If the 'shifting sand effect' is to be avoided, then real change must be owned by those who use it. Ownership of the change process and its

results must be the prerogative of those who are doing the work. By owning the change, the staff come to feel it is their decision. It is their property. We tend to cherish, care for, and preserve those things which we ourselves have created.

The new norms and values which come to pass in the situation where change has occurred are far more likely to remain permanent if the staff themselves feel they have created them. Such a process requires a skilful change agent who helps them to produce change from the 'bottom-up', thereby avoiding the pitfalls of 'top-down' change.

A 'bottom-up' change strategy

As has been suggested, it is possible to bring about change in people's behaviour by a direct authoritarian 'power–coercive' approach, i.e., by telling them how to do things differently. Rogers' (1969) influential philosophy, however, suggests that there are risks in this model. When the authority moves on, or becomes less effective, then there is a danger that a reversion to old norms and values takes place. Change can only become permanent if the desired values and attitudes have become a permanent part of the people in the care setting. An institutional framework can be broken down, but an alternative resilient framework must take its place if the changes are not to be swept away when the change agent departs. For alternative goals and values to be reached – for people to come to a different view of their world – a more egalitarian strategy is a necessary tool. Lewin's (1958) classic change theory defines 'no change' as a 'quasi-stationary equilibrium . . . a state comparable to that of a river which flows with a given velocity in a given direction during a certain time interval'. He describes social changes as comparable to a change in the velocity and the direction of that river, and sees the change process as having three basic steps:

Unfreezing – when the motivation to create some sort of change occurs, the impetus for this coming from three possible mechanisms:
a) *Lack of confirmation or disconfirmation*, i.e., the awareness of a need for change because expectations have not been met.
b) *Induction of guilt or anxiety*, i.e., uncomfortable feelings because of some action or lack of action.
c) *Psychological safety* when a former obstacle to change has been removed.

Moving – when change is planned and initiated where cognitive redefinition occurs to look at the problem from a new perspective either through 'identification' or 'scanning' (the former solution provided by a knowledgeable peer: the latter solution found in a variety of sources).

Refreezing – when change is integrated into the value system and stabilised into a new equilibrium.

In order to 'unfreeze' existing norms and 'move' the staff to 'refreeze' into new norms, a tool to do the job is required. Many alternatives are available, and producing change in nursing is often a designated role for many practitioners, managers and educators. The idea of embodying change strategies in a specifically designated person, the change agent, to produce change is accepted by many authors on the subject (Rogers, 1969; and Lewin, 1958 among them).

Ottaway (1976; 1980) identifies a change strategy using a change agent, with the ability to use Lewin's model, who can work to implement change from the 'bottom-up'. He identifies a strategy where managers and educators act in support roles to the on site change agent, who, in this instance, works with staff and patients over a period of time (it may take many years!) to produce change (Fig. 3.3).

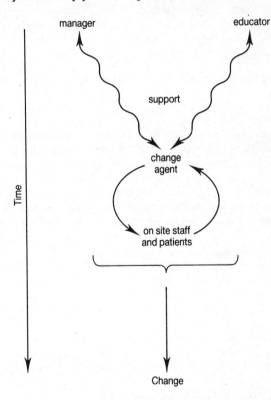

Fig. 3.3 'Bottom up' change strategy.

Clearly, if any one element in this model is lacking, then the chances of success are hindered if not blocked completely, e.g., the manager is unsupported.

Ottaway (1976) identifies six crucial factors for this type of change.

- Bottom up – there is participation of the 'shopfloor' workers and the change may move up into the rest of the organisation rather than the reverse.
- Pilot site – the new norms are practiced here first rather than across the whole organisation at once. A site is chosen where the staff are willing to participate.
- Training follows change – participator begins to feel need for new knowledge and skill which is then supplied rather than trying to change people for new skills and expecting them to apply them.
- Contracting – the staff decide on the how, what, and when of the change for their own small unit.
- Made to order – the change process is fitted to the unique individual setting and not applied as a preplanned package everywhere.
- Felt need – the change is determined by the needs the staff feel, rather than imposed by outsiders.

These key elements are incorporated into various steps of the change process.

Step 1   Agreeing goals
The staff get together and agree new goals and directions, however large or small they may be. What are we trying to do? How can we improve things? The skills of the change agent are seen as instrumental in guiding the ideas and generating questions, without seeming to impose plans. The person may, for example, be a ward sister, but the important features are that they have knowledge and skill, work on site with the staff, and are seen to be part of the team without necessarily directing it.

Step 2   Make a diagnosis
How is the work organised? What is wrong? What are the aims of the organisation or unit? What are each staff member's abilities? What resources are available? What is the management style like? In other words, the change agent assesses the nature of the organisation in order to make a plan of action.

Step 3   The design of intervention
This should be done by the people who have to make it work and they should map out what will be changed, how it will be done, and even how long.

Step 4   Implement the intervention
Put the plans into action, and have review sessions as matters progress.

Step 5   Skill training
Enable the staff to learn the new skills which they begin to feel they need, e.g., better communication skills, more knowledge on a nursing problem, how to use a computer, etc.

Step 6   Reinforce new norms
Talk about success and congratulate each other! Give praise when it is due and be wary of criticism. Rewards might be offered, e.g., study leave, bursaries, etc.

Step 7   Replicating
Transferring the experience and knowledge and repeating the steps on other sites.

> *Example*
> A nurse on a unit wishes to implement primary nursing in her setting. At a staff meeting she mentions the subject (Who is interested? Who isn't?) and gets the staff thinking about it. Some agree it is a goal they would like to learn more about. A few more meetings take place (often at the pub or someone's home – it is often difficult to confer a meeting at work!) including meetings with the night staff. (Step 1).
>
> The aims and the problems are discussed. Currently, care seems a little impersonal, sometimes less organised. The theory of primary nursing looks like it might help solve these. (Step 2).
>
> Plans are drawn up for allocating patients, agreeing case loads, who will be a primary nurse, who an associate. The organisation of the ward is reviewed, and an experimental implementation period of six months agreed. (Step 3).
>
> A date is decided to begin primary nursing. Weekly meetings are held to review difficulties, as well as informal discussion sessions at each shift change, as need arises. Problems are reviewed, case loads adjusted, grievances aired. (Step 4).
>
> The staff find they need to know more. Lectures on accountability, visits to other units, meetings with other primary nurses are requested. More books and literature are obtained. (Step 5).
>
> Things seem to be progressing. The staff say they enjoy the new sense of responsibility and sister is more free to support the staff. Patients like having 'my nurse', and say so. The manager notices the happy atmosphere on the ward and compliments the staff. Relatives praise it. Complimentary letters are received. (Step 6).
>
> Some staff move to other areas to pass on their ideas. Other staff come to the unit to seek advice and return to their own areas to try it out themselves. (Step 7).

For simplicity, each of the steps has been reduced, but, as may be seen, they are highly complex acts, fraught with difficulties. The change process is rarely so linear and logical, and this theory will be explored in more detail in the proceeding chapters.

In effect, the application of Ottaway's strategy is a call to 'proletarianise' (Bond, 1978) the process of change in nursing. The avoidance of this 'top down' authoritarian approach encompasses the transfer of the government of change into the hands of those whose lives are most affected by it. The 'pedagogic dialogue' (Freire, 1973) which takes place between change agent and the on site staff is seen as crucial in generating ideas and changing old norms into new ones. The staff are helped to become aware of their situation and guided in the transition to alternative methods. In so doing, they own their change process and, therefore, have an investment in its success and retention.

References

Benner, P. (1984). *From Novice to Expert*. Addison Wesley, California.

Beyers, M. and Phillips, C. (1971). *Nursing Management for Patient Care*. Little, Brown, Boston.

Bond, S. (1978). *Dilemmas in Clinical Research*. Paper presented at Northern Regional Health Authority Seminar on Developments in Nursing. Unpublished.

Clarke, M. (1978). Getting through the work. *In* Dingwall, R. and McIntosh, J. (Eds), *Readings in the Sociology of Nursing*. Churchill Livingstone, Edinburgh.

Freire, P. (1973). *Pedagogy of the Oppressed*. Writers and Readers Publishing Cooperative, London.

Gibbs, J., Evans, M. and Redway, S. (1987). *The Report of the Enquiry into Nye Bevan Lodge*. Unpublished. DHSS.

Goffman, I. (1961). *Asylums*. Penguin, Harmondsworth.

Lenara, V. (1984). *Heroism as a Nursing Value*. Sisterhood Evniki, Athens.

Lewin, K. (1958). The group reason and social change. *In* Maccoby, E. (Ed), *Readings in Social Psychology*. Holt, Rinehart and Winston, London.

Macdonald, B. and Rich, C. (1984). *Look Me in the Eye*. Women's Press, London.

Martin, J. and Evans, D. (1984). *Hospitals in Trouble*. Blackwell, Oxford.

Ottaway, R. N. (1976). A change strategy to implement new norms, new style and new environments in the work organisation. *Personnel Review*, 5 (1), 13–15.

Ottaway, R. N. (1980). *Defining the Change Agent*. Unpublished research paper. University of Manchester Institute of Technology, Department of Management Sciences, Manchester.

Rogers, C. (1969). *Freedom to Learn*. Merrill, Columbus, Ohio.

Rogers, E. M. (1962). *Diffusion of Innovations*. Free Press, New York.

Salvage, J. (1988). *Facilitating Model Based Nursing*. Unpublished paper given at Gateshead School of Nursing Models Conference.

Scheff, T. (1967). *Mental Illness and Social Processes*. Harper and Row, London.

Yorkshire Television (1986). *The Granny Business*.

4

The change obstacle course: additional perspectives on the change process

'It is often safer to be in chains, than to be free.'
Franz Kafka   *Metamorphosis*

Kafka's phrase is a salutory reminder to nurses of the dangers of change – both to themselves as individuals and as a group. As the previous chapter has suggested, not everyone approaches change with the same degree of energy and commitment. Using the problem-solving framework can help in organising change, but rarely does it work so neatly or in such a linear fashion. Nurses and the world they work in are far too contingent.

Many nurses in many settings have tried to change what goes on around them, only to find their energy dissipated and their enthusiasm burnt out when confronted with the killing tripartite; obstructive management, unsupportive educators and resistant colleagues. Under these circumstances, it is little wonder that many keen and committed nurses have given up in despair and resentment. They discover that 'when you stop banging your head against a brick wall, the headache goes away'!

Change is difficult, if not impossible – as many nurses have found to their cost, when they have decided to 'go it alone', or have been thrust in by the management of the institution to an undesirable setting to sort things out. Georgiades and Phillimore (1975) illustrated how the 'hero innovator' is not as effective a change agent as is often assumed. When used by the organisation to put things to rights they may exhaust themselves, may move on leaving things to revert to the status quo, or they may fail and become discredited. In the process, they discredit the change process and reinforce the view that it is impossible to change the situation anyway.

The culture of change

Toffler (1973) writes of the 'death of permanence'. We live in a society where everything is open to question and threatened by change and, moreover, where such change is accelerating. The health care system cannot remain isolated from this, nor can its nurses. The health services themselves must now accept a new culture (the status quo is not an option), and this requires that change, the acceptance of it and the practice of it, must be part of the normal day-to-day activities of the organisation. The acceptance of this new culture has not occurred wholesale or simultaneously in the various levels of the health services. There is a risk to nurses, as individuals or in small groups, who seek to change things in their setting when other parts of the organisation are stuck in the preservation of the existing order mould. Changing practice at clinical level has difficulty in expanding and progressing if the total organisation has not accepted the culture of change. It does not render change impossible, but it does produce limitations. The change agent must be aware of these factors in order to limit the obstruction they can present, limit the damage that can be done, and how to overcome or get around them.

Praill and Baldwin (1988) note that 'Rather than the continuation of frenetic, isolated and disjointed clinical practice and innovation attempts, a system is required which is itself innovative. Responsibility for innovation should be corporate, rather than invested in key individuals'. They suggest, like Toffler (1973), that change itself needs to be an inherent part of the total system on which nurses work.

Futhermore, nurses must not expect that they or other professions can be the sole determinants of change. Many innovations blowing through the NHS are led not by those who work in it, but are a product of rising demands and expectations of the consumer. Indeed, this is seen as preferable; 'A structure is required to facilitate the development of active consumer-led systems, which demand change for the benefit of client groups' (Praill and Baldwin, 1988). If this is the case, then where do nurses fit into this scheme of things? They are providers of care (and therefore must respond to consumer-led demand). Yet, in some respects, they are also consumers – either as potential patients themselves, or of the workplace which provides them with a living, as well as (hopefully) job satisfaction.

If the recent trend towards primary nursing in the UK is taken as an example, whence comes the push for change? There seems to be a double-edged blade at work, but which came first, or whether both arrived in tandem, it is difficult to discern.

Patients as consumers demand
more personal care, more information,
more accountability from care providers.

Nurses' professional aspirations,
dissatisfaction with less
personal modes of care, more
control over individual patient care.

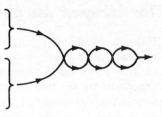

Perhaps the culture of change in health care is at its most potent and most successful when the needs of both provider and recipient have shared aspirations. There seems little doubt that such innovation is most successfully accomplished in a climate which encourages it, that is, when the system in which nurses work has accepted that change is an inevitable and desirable part of its culture. The organisation as a whole benefits from this too. It seems, for example, that the desire to remain 'in chains' is a response to the threat of change and all the upset it can bring. Studies have shown, however, (Orton, 1981; McClure *et al.*, 1983; Price Waterhouse, 1988) that working climates where staff feel they are supported, where they feel they are learning, and where they feel they *can* innovate, are more likely not only to recruit nurses, but to retain them as well. 'Indeed, what does come through rather vividly from the data is that magnet hospitals have the total picture in place: the management is supportive of professional nursing practice within the context of a teaching/learning environment' (McClure *et al.*, 1983).

It appears that the ideal climate for nurses, those they serve, the organisation in which they work, and those who manage it, is achieved in a setting where innovation is the norm. Nurses in such a setting are not necessarily seeking and using power for power's sake, rather they feel that they are not powerless. Being involved, feeling listened to, knowing that management is responsive and not oppressive, appear to be important feelings to nurses which support them in their work and make them feel free of their chains to innovate. However, it may be wondered how many nurses today work in a climate such as this. Perhaps not the majority, many might answer, although Toffler (1973) appears to offer some hope in his model. The 'accelerative thrust' of change will eventually overwhelm all institutions which fail to respond to the needs of their workers and their consumers. Like the incidence of Canute against the waves, the tide cannot be held back. Sadly, because change in some areas lags behind that in others, some nurses might have to wait a little longer and struggle a little harder for their professional aspirations to be realised.

The conspiracy of nurses

If the nurse as a change agent cannot change things alone, then he or she must enter a conspiracy. The word 'conspire' has its origins in the Latin (*con* – together; *spīrāre* – to breathe). To conspire requires groups of nurses and others to come together in a shared under-standing and common purpose. In so doing, they have more strength to overcome obstacles, they can share and develop new knowledge, and can draw support from each other. Using the models of Rogers and Ottoway sited in the previous chapter, an example would be of the change generation and change adopter on one unit reinforcing one another to overcome influence of the laggards.

> *Example*
> 'We got together (myself and the two ENs) to see what we could do about them. There were three in particular. Every time they got together on the off duty things seemed to get more difficult. They seemed to undermine what we wanted to do. I don't mind admitting that we plotted. The simple logic of managing the off duty so that they never got together worked wonderfully.' (Ward Sister.)

Introducing new norms into a setting is about getting everyone to take on board these values. In some instances, division of the opposi-tion may accelerate the process! However, working together towards shared goals is both rewarding and more likely to produce success as the rabbits in *Watership Down* (Adams, 1972), or the comrades of *The Hobbit* (Tolkien, 1966) discovered.

Resistance

Conspiracy may help to overcome the resistance to change, but a more potent weapon is knowledge. Resistance initially has its roots in fear – fear of doing things differently, of losing privileges, of feeling inade-quate or ignorant. Managers can feel threatened, for example, when staff undertake things they do not know about, while others can resist new practices because they do not understand them.

Giving staff the knowledge of who they are, what goals they are aiming for, and how they can achieve them, is an important part of the process. Some of these aspects are dealt with in the test and the case study (Chapter 6) emphasising the need to 'get people together' so that ideas, knowledge, fears and hopes can be shared. This incorporates a wide ranging programme of staff development, teaching and promoting self-awareness. It includes the use of many educational strategies; from providing library facilities, courses and conferences, to workshops on communication skills. Pearson (1985), for example, has explored the use of drama in attitude changes in the Oxford Nursing Development Units, along with a variety of other strategies. Purdy *et al.*, (1988) detail a similar process in the Tameside Nursing Development Unit. It may also reduce resistance, reassuring staff that the planned change will not bring redeployment or redundancies, for example, or, if this is likely, providing information about staff protection.

> *Example*
> 'The boss looked horrified when I mentioned that I was thinking of letting the patients have access to the nursing notes. I spent quite a few weeks giving him information, talking it through, so that he fully understood the reasoning behind it and the prospects: I didn't make a move in that direction until I felt sure he understood it all and would support me.'
> (Charge nurse in a community unit.)

Any nurse who has tried to innovate will probably have encountered many of the classic comments offered to resist change:

> We've been doing it like that for years!
> I'm too old to change!
> The patients wouldn't like it!
> We've done it before and it didn't work!
> We haven't got the money/staff/time!
> It's not that simple!
> But we work in the real world!

Exasperation when encountering such remarks is common and, in retrospect, may be humourous. However, they are signs of the very real fears that colleagues can have about change. These fears can only be overcome through:

> education – providing staff with the knowledge and skills they need to do things differently
> time – letting people 'unfreeze, move and refreeze' at their own pace (see Chapter 3)
> reinforcement – using praise when it's due when success, however minor, is achieved

Resistance, however, may take more sinister forms than mumbled procrastination. It may, in extremes, move into open hostility, resentment and anger. It may produce conflicts with colleagues other than nurses (witness, for example, the reaction of some medical staff when nurses have refused to help with ECT (electroconvulsive therapy)). In addition, it may put the person pushing for change in conflict with the organisation in which he/she works, e.g., the effects on the 'whistle blowers' in big mental institutions (Martin, 1984), or with their professional bodies and staff organisations. Anyone entering the process of change needs to have a clear understanding of their professional boundaries and accountability. The risks to the individual under such extreme circumstances cannot be overemphasised, although they appear to be relatively rare.

For most nurses day-to-day change at clinical level rarely comes into the category of some of those which hit the headlines. It is more likely to be characterised by the daily frustrations of petty obstacles and gnawing frustrations. Planned change is therefore essential to minimise the conflicts which can occur (see Chapter 5).

Planned change – additional dimensions

The change process, as described in the previous chapter, is a fairly linear and logical series of steps. This provides us with a framework for planning and implementing change, but is cannot cover all eventualities. In reality, the 'human element' can defy the most rational of processes, adding new complexities and uncertainties. Turrill (1985) identifies seven factors which change agents must consider:

* *Agreeing the core purposes of the organisation* – setting the philosophy or statement of mission which makes explicit 'why we are all here' and 'what we want to achieve'.
* *Sharing a vision of a better future* – enough colleagues have to share the same vision of the aims of the change which may be years ahead.
* *Operating principles* – setting out the values, what is important and what is not, to help guide the nurse when faced with uncertainties.
* *Mapping the environment* – identifying the implications for change on other groups and working out where resistance might come from.
* *Transition management* – working out how you will manage the journey from where you are to where you want to be in the change process.
* *Resistance reduction* – working with power groupings/individuals maintaining communication.
* *Seeking commitment* – winning people over, identifying key groups and individuals.

Example

In our unit we believe that every patient has the right to choice in his care.	= Agreeing the core purpose of the organisation.
We want to provide choices at mealtimes, move away from rigid routines, give access to nursing and medical notes.	= Sharing a vision of a better future.
No patient will have any treatment or care without first being given the opportunity for informed consent.	= Operating principles.
Consider the implications of the code of conduct, maintaining confidentiality, possible conflicts with management, doctors.	= Mapping the environment.
Set up a working group to study the opportunities. One person to research and document progress. Develop new nursing notes.	= Transition management.
Meet with managers, doctors, colleagues. Discuss with relatives and patients. Provide written information.	= Resistance reduction.
Offer staff development programme, teaching, study days, improve job satisfaction.	= Seeking.

This chapter has explored a number of additional themes in relation to the change process. While various models and strategies may offer us a logical framework for action, the reality of change, as has been suggested, is rarely so smooth and linear. Any nurse setting out on the path of change is taking a journey into the unknown to some extent. The ideas discussed so far have sought to provide a map to help with the route; but help is all they can do. That is what can make change so exciting and stimulating. When all the factors have been thought through, planned and practiced, in the end there is still an element of adventure, of exploration. In using the logical process of change, it is also necessary to accept the element of the intuitive. The former is the scientific component, the latter the artistic. In the change process, both are necessary parts!

While the 'hero innovator' is a questionable myth, what cannot be underestimated is the real courage needed by *all* nurses who undertake change. In that sense, all nurses who act as change agents are heroes or heroines. Heroism is not just found in the grand acts of history, it is also found in every nurse who attempts to overcome difficulties, however small. As Lenara (1981) notes: 'The goal of the hero and the goal of the nurse coincide. The goal of the hero is to transcend what threatens. And the goal of the nurse is to transcend the obstacles which emerge, from outside and within herself, to threaten her nursing ideal'.

References

Adams, R. (1972). *Watership Down*. Puffin, London.

Georgiades, N. J. and Phillimore, L. (1975).The myth of the hero innovator. *In* Kiernan, C. C. and Woodford, F. P. (Eds), *Behaviour Modification with the Severely Retarded*. Associated Scientific Publications, London.

Lenara, V. (1981). *Heroism as a Nursing Value*. Sisterhood Evniki, Athens.

Martin, J. P. (1984). *Hospitals in Trouble*. Blackwell, Oxford.

McClure, M. L., Poulin, M. A., Sovie, M. D., Wandelt, M. A. (1983). *Magnet Hospitals: Attraction and Retention of Professional Nurses*. American Academy of Nursing, Kansas City.

Orton, H. (1981). *The Ward Learning Climate and Student Nurse Response*. Royal College of Nursing, London.

Pearson, A. (1985). *The Effects of Introducing New Norms in a Nursing Unit: An Analysis of the Process of Change*. Unpublished PhD Thesis, University of London.

Praill, T. and Baldwin, S. (1988). Beyond hero-innovation: real change in unreal systems. *Behavioural Psychotherapy*,16, 1–14.

Price Waterhouse (1988). *Nurse Recruitment and Retention*. Price Waterhouse, London.

Purdy, E., Wright, S. G. and Johnson M. L. (1988). Change for the better. *Nursing Times*, 84 (38), 34–5.

Toffler, A. (1973). *Future Shock*. Pan Books, London.

Tolkien, J. R. R. (1966). *The Hobbit*. Unwin Books, London.

Turrill, T. (1988). Change and innovation. *A Challenge for the NHS*. Management Series 10. Institute of Health Services Management, London.

5

Costs and conflicts

'(Wilde was to be charged a large fee for an operation.) "Ah, well then," said Oscar, "I suppose that I shall have to die beyond my means." '

R. H. Sherard   *Life of Oscar Wilde*

Resources required to meet change cover a wide area, but one which immediately comes to mind is that of finance, probably because it always seems to be the greatest battle and loudest niggle within the service. However, other aspects need to be considered such as the effects on the personnel involved, including the change agent and all the others affected by the change process.

Stresses and strains on the staff

The cost to individuals can be far-reaching, and is identifiable in both positive and negative terms. Innovators are, by nature of their pursuit, faced with many stresses; the first being how to approach the challenge of change to achieve success, and yet minimise the personal conflicts. Thomsom (1977) identifies that over-anxiety resulting in annoyance or anger can detract objectivity and concentration. He also suggests that 'indifference, half-heartedness, over-confidence, are equally disturbing: persistence and appreciation can only come from a certain degree of interest and concern. A moderate but effective motivation is needed'. Each individual will have to appraise themselves to identify and recognise the point at which they need to switch off (even if it be for a short period) and perhaps withdraw from the situation in order to maintain their physical, psychological and emotional well-being.

Stress can manifest itself in many ways. The change agent must recognise signs and symptoms of stress in themselves and adopt strategies to overcome these in order that he/she doesn't reach burnout, and also the change agent must recognise signs of stress in the target group and intervene when and where appropriate.

Cooper *et al.* (1988) have identified the major symptoms of stress and these can be summarised under three main headings.

Table 5.1 Major symptoms of stress (after Cooper et al., 1988).

Physical symptoms of stress	Mental symptoms of stress	Stress related ailments
Lack of appetite	Constant irritability with people	Hypertension: high blood pressure
Craving for food when under pressure	Feeling unable to cope	Coronary thrombosis: heart attack
Frequent indigestion or heartburn	Lack of interest in life	Migraine
Constipation or diarrhoea	Constant or recurrent fear of disease	Hay fever and allergies
Insomnia	A feeling of being a failure	Asthma
Constant tiredness	A feeling of being bad or of self-hatred	Pruritus: intense itching
Tendency to sweat for no good reason	Difficulty in making decisions	Peptic ulcers
Nervous twitches	A feeling of ugliness	Constipation
Nail-biting	Loss of interest in other people	Colitis
Headaches	Awareness of suppressed anger	Menstrual difficulties
Cramps and muscle spasms	Inability to show true feelings	Nervous dyspepsia: flatulence and indigestion
Nausea	A feeling of being the target of other people's animosity	Overactive thyroid gland
Breathlessness without exertion	Loss of sense of humour	Diabetes mellitus
Fainting spells	Feeling of neglect	Skin disorders
Frequent crying or desire to cry	Dread of the future	Tuberculosis
Impotence or frigidity	A feeling of having failed as a person or parent	Depression
Inability to sit still without fidgeting	A feeling of having no confidence	
High blood pressure	Difficulty in concentrating	
	The inability to finish one task before rushing on to the next	
	An intense fear of open or enclosed spaces or of being alone	

Each individual appraises the stressfulness of a situation uniquely; the view, opinions, emotions and circumstances all have a bearing on the way we think and feel about ourselves. Bailey (1985) summarises that stress results from:

'The way we think about ourselves and our circumstances.
The meaning we give to the demands we consider are being made on us.
The value we put on the importance of caring for others.'

The psychologist Chernis (1980) has suggested that burnout is a type of disease as a result of overcommitment, and later suggested that burnout meant the 'withdrawal from work in response to excessive stress or dissatisfaction'. Lazarus and Lannier (1978) define coping as 'an individual's attempt to manage (to master, tolerate, reduce, minimise, etc.) internal and external environmental demands or conflicts which tax one's resources'.

One of the first attempts at coping with stress is recognising that it exists. Change agents in leadership positions need to have sufficient awareness to recognise it in themselves, but, when they do not, this is the point where the supportive managers or colleagues should step in. The change agent needs also to be able to recognise stress effects on others. Stress which produces the kind of negative effects (as opposed to the positive ones of stimulation and motivation at work) as listed above is a sign that things are going wrong.

Does the change agent lack the skills or knowledge to do the job?
Are they expecting too much of themselves too quickly?
Are the resources inadequate to meet the change requirements?
Are the support methods failing (e.g., has the support from managers or colleagues dissipated)?

It may mean that stress on the change agents and their colleagues can put the whole change process into question. There has been a tendency in nursing to find a scapegoat when things go wrong. It is too easy to focus, for example, on the change agent. Salvage (1988) notes that when nurses complain that they cannot cope, the nurse is often held to blame, instead of examining the situation which has produced the failure to cope.

A full discussion on the subject of stress is beyond the scope of this text, but it needs to be recognised that stress is an inevitable part of the change process. Stress may produce either positive or negative effects on the staff, depending upon its degree of intensity. The stress usually arises not because of any failings in the change agents or their colleagues, rather as a result of problems with the planning or carrying through of the change process. Some points to consider to alleviate the situation include:

- Review the whole change process using the Ottoway (1976) and Turrill (1985) models. Was a factor not identified in the planning stage? Are the reviews not frequent enough? Is there greater pressure than anticipated from resisters?
- Adjust the change process and replan in the light of new difficulties.
- Examine the roles that the staff occupy as these can be a source of stress (Harding and Conway, 1978). Are they experiencing role overload (through having too much to do) or role conflict (different role expectations between the person on a job and those they work with, families, friends and so on)? The end result of either difficulty is role strain, when the stress manifests itself in the kind of physiological and psychological symptoms mentioned by Cooper *et al.* (1988).
- Identify weaknesses in the knowledge or skill of the staff which are producing role fulfilment difficulties. Provide education to fill the gap.
- Provide counselling, assertiveness training, stress awareness training or relaxable techniques for staff who are experiencing difficulties as appropriate. Within the NHS, these facilities are not always available, but there has been a growing trend in recent years to develop counselling skills for key staff and to provide a counselling service in many settings. Many colleges, schools of nursing and other educational institutions provide courses in self-awareness and assertiveness and relaxation techniques. Other staff organisations, such as the Royal College of Nursing, also provide these, along with an independent counselling service.

Under these circumstances, it might be seen that the change process might also be a personal growth experience for those who are going through it. It must also be remembered that stressful situations at work can be exacerbated if the person is also experiencing stress in their non-working lives.

Cooper *et al.*'s (1988) stress inventory gives an indication of the extent of the issue (Table 5.2).

If the staff and the change agents are experiencing stress, there is also a moral obligation on those who support them to examine their role. Is the education and management support that is needed being offered? Are the resources being provided? Are sufficient staff available? It is important to look at the individual's coping abilities and find ways to enhance them if stress occurs. It is also important to ensure that the situation in which the change agent and his/her colleagues must work is examined for flaws. Individuals may have weaknesses, but so do the circumstances in which they are required to work.

Table 5.2 The life stress inventory (after Cooper *et al.*, 1988).

Place a cross (x) in the 'Yes' column for each event which has taken place in the last two years. Circle a number on the scale which best describes how upsetting the event was to you, e.g., 10 for death of spouse.

Event	Yes	Scale
Bought house		1 2 3 4 5 6 7 8 9 10
Sold house		1 2 3 4 5 6 7 8 9 10
Moved house		1 2 3 4 5 6 7 8 9 10
Major house renovation		1 2 3 4 5 6 7 8 9 10
Increased or new bank loan/mortgage		1 2 3 4 5 6 7 8 9 10
Separation from loved one		1 2 3 4 5 6 7 8 9 10
End of relationship		1 2 3 4 5 6 7 8 9 10
Got engaged		1 2 3 4 5 6 7 8 9 10
Got married		1 2 3 4 5 6 7 8 9 10
Marital problem		1 2 3 4 5 6 7 8 9 10
Awaiting divorce		1 2 3 4 5 6 7 8 9 10
Divorce		1 2 3 4 5 6 7 8 9 10
Child started school/nursery		1 2 3 4 5 6 7 8 9 10
Increased nursing responsibilities for elderly or sick person		1 2 3 4 5 6 7 8 9 10
Problems with relatives		1 2 3 4 5 6 7 8 9 10
Problems with friends/neighbours		1 2 3 4 5 6 7 8 9 10
Pet-related problems		1 2 3 4 5 6 7 8 9 10
Work-related problems		1 2 3 4 5 6 7 8 9 10
Change in nature of work		1 2 3 4 5 6 7 8 9 10
Threat of redundancy		1 2 3 4 5 6 7 8 9 10
Changed job		1 2 3 4 5 6 7 8 9 10
Made redundant		1 2 3 4 5 6 7 8 9 10
Unemployed		1 2 3 4 5 6 7 8 9 10
Retired		1 2 3 4 5 6 7 8 9 10
Financial difficulty		1 2 3 4 5 6 7 8 9 10
Insurance problem		1 2 3 4 5 6 7 8 9 10
Legal problem		1 2 3 4 5 6 7 8 9 10
Emotional or physical illness of close family or relative		1 2 3 4 5 6 7 8 9 10
Serious illness of close family or relative requiring hospitalisation		1 2 3 4 5 6 7 8 9 10
Surgical operation experienced by family member or relative		1 2 3 4 5 6 7 8 9 10
Death of spouse		1 2 3 4 5 6 7 8 9 10
Death of family member or relative		1 2 3 4 5 6 7 8 9 10

table continued

Table 5.2 *continued*

Event	Yes	Scale
Death of close friend		1 2 3 4 5 6 7 8 9 10
Emotional or physical illness of yourself		1 2 3 4 5 6 7 8 9 10
Serious illness requiring your own hospitalisation		1 2 3 4 5 6 7 8 9 10
Surgical operation on yourself		1 2 3 4 5 6 7 8 9 10
Pregnancy		1 2 3 4 5 6 7 8 9 10
Birth of baby		1 2 3 4 5 6 7 8 9 10
Birth of grandchild		1 2 3 4 5 6 7 8 9 10
Family member left home		1 2 3 4 5 6 7 8 9 10
Difficult relationship with children		1 2 3 4 5 6 7 8 9 10
Difficult relationship with parents		1 2 3 4 5 6 7 8 9 10

Plot total score below

Low stress		High stress
1	50	100

Case study 1

Sister Smith, whilst extremely experienced in her speciality, was new to the health authority and to the ward to which she had been appointed. During the first few weeks of her appointment she observed the daily and weekly happenings and events of the ward.

Tuesday mornings and Thursday afternoons seemed to present an atmosphere of anxiety, organisation beyond that which was normal, and a degree of apprehension within the ward. These were the times of the consultants' ward rounds. Not only was the ward organised and spotless, but no visitors were allowed in and the patients had to sit neatly on their beds, irrespective of their needs, until after the great event. Even going to the toilet had to wait until after!

Sister Smith was not happy that her patients' days were being disrupted in this way. The ward comprised long stay and rehabilitation elderly patients in the main, few were acute admissions. The two rounds were for different consultants, so there were always patients who would not be seen on at least one of these sessions.

Observation of the ritual of the 'ward round' revealed that neither consultants had time for the long stay patients, walking past them with only a wave, and only a fraction of the time for those undergoing rehabilitation, but a good deal of time was spent with those patients who had been acute admissions or were 'interesting cases'.

The effect of this organisation was that staff resources were not being utilised fully; therapy time was being wasted, and patients were not receiving the style of care which was conducive to maintaining or achieving their optimum levels of achievement. Indeed, the only people who really liked the arrangement were the consultants!

Sister Smith, having gained support from the nursing staff, defined a new approach to the 'ward round'. All new admissions, acute and critically ill patients were prepared for the consultant to see and examine them. At the start, the nurse taking the round would go through that particular consultant's patients and together they would identify any others which required to be seen for a specific reason. These patients would then be prepared in the manner appropriate, whilst the 'ward round' commenced. The remaining patients who the consultant did not feel he needed to see carried on with therapies, treatments, or their original activities. The consultant went to them during the round to say hello as a matter of courtesy, causing as little disruption to their normal activities as possible.

The consultants took a long time to adjust to the new organisation of 'the ward round'. Comments such as, 'I don't know who is who', and, 'I like them all on their beds' were voiced for some time. The staff were much happier, as were the patients, and, despite the consultants' superior attitude and threats, Sister Smith stood her ground, suggesting that if they objected to her organisation they should see the unit managers!

Sister knew that her case was founded on good operational and organisational strategy and not on a power–coercive, ego-boosting strategy, which she suspected was the case of the medical staff.

Another conflict which was overcome by this change in organisation was that the patients who were not receiving a visit from the consultants stopped feeling as though they were unimportant. They were busy doing other things which were to their benefit, and this they recognised.

This case study demonstrates how a small and simple area of change can cause conflict. The conflict being founded not on what is best for the recipients, but on maintaining the status quo to preserve the individual's power. The combined result of nurses acting together and management support was essential to ride out the conflict and confront the consultants. This conflict was anticipated, met and dealt with.

An area where interpersonal conflict is occasionally encountered is between the health care workers and the patient/client. The public today are becoming much better informed, through education and the media, and are demanding that they be involved in the discussions and decisions made about themselves and their families. As professionals, health care workers are taught to assume they have more knowledge and power than their patient/client. Many nurses feel unable to cope with the stress of the new kind of relationship which emerges with the patient. Task allocation, Menzies (1960) has argued, allowed nurses to hide from the stress of a closer relationship with the patient and his problems. If the tasks, for example, which nurses have used as a coping strategy are removed, what are they replaced with? It is necessary to return to the point made earlier:

Education so that staff feel equipped to cope with a new way of doing things.

Support from colleagues, and an atmosphere where both praise and sympathy are given freely, where feelings can be easily talked about, exchanged and understood.

When confronted with change at clinical level, Salvage (1988) suggests that nurses go through changes not unlike the grieving process:

Shock is the first likely response; people facing change feel threatened, overwhelmed, anxious and panicky. As we know from research on patients, fear tends to close down your communication channels and limit your rational faculties.

Defensive retreat can follow from an inability to cope with this shock; it is a kind of denial of it. People become negative and withdrawn, or occasionally falsely optimistic and euphoric.

Acknowledgement, as in bereavement, is an important step towards acceptance, but it can involve apathy and a nostalgia for the good old days and ways – just as we tend to remember the dead person in a favourable light.

Adaptation occurs if these preceding stages are worked through. When the nurse begins to mobilise her resources and abilities to meet the new situation, she begins to learn: now comes a time of challenge and growth.

(Salvage, 1988)

With the support of the kind discussed so far in this chapter, the conflicts for staff in the change process can be minimised. The change agents and their colleagues can experience the process as a benefit not only to their client, but as a time of challenge and growth for themselves as well.

Staff changes

The implications for changing the norms and style of the workplace cannot be underestimated. Where change is minor, the effects can be minimal, but change on a grander scale – such as the wholesale shifting of a group's philosophy and approach to work (for example, in shifting from an institutionalised to a personalised model of care) – can produce quite dramatic effects. Ultimately, some staff will not feel able to work with the new style and, as Ottoway (1976), Martin (1984) and Wright (1985) have suggested, they may leave. While the departure of some staff may be a cause for concern (it may cost more to recruit new staff), there are several aspects to this problem. Firstly, it must be questioned whether or not it is desirable that they have left. To be blunt, is the organisation better off without them? Were they so resistant to change that it would simply not have been cost-effective to pour resources and energy into persuading them to participate? Secondly, did they leave because the change strategy was wrong and, if so, is it that which needs to be examined? Thirdly, is their leaving a cause for concern because they were considered to be among the 'better' staff? If this is the case, it may be that their qualities were overestimated, or it may be that the change has taken a new path and is not perhaps producing a change for the better.

There is a value judgement being made here, for it is assumed that change which produces a more personalised climate for both staff and patients is 'better'. There is, of course, an opposing perspective to this. The staff who have got used to the more institutionalised approach (as depicted so succinctly in Martin (1984)) may not see the new approach as 'better' but 'worse' because of the loss of the status quo, the old power structures, and their privileges.

In part, it is up to the reader to make their own value judgements on these issues. However, in the final analysis, what nurses want is of secondary importance to what patients or clients want. If nurses believe that they know so much better than the patient or client, then the obligation is up to nursing to explain its case to the consumer so that he or she can make an informed choice. Certainly, if the mass of evidence that has accumulated over the years is anything to go by, patients are fairly clear about what they want from nurses – a service that is humane, friendly, informative and personal, and takes full account of their needs, and does not seek to fit them into someone else's roles. At the last, it is the patient who judges.

The client's perceptions

Almost all changes at clinical level will affect the recipient of care. In this respect, he or she provides the ultimate test of the change. The change process has to be 'sold' to the client as well as the staff. It seems that many complaints in care (DHSS, 1984–87) can be attributed to the failure of the professionals to communicate adequately about why they do what they do with patients.

Example

A family complain to the community nurse who has been helping their relative, a young woman, at home. She is disabled after a road accident, but the nurse is trying to encourage her independence by allowing her to feed herself and teaching her to do things for herself. The relatives see this as 'uncaring' as they think everything should be 'done for' their loved one. The nurse has not 'sold' her style of care to the relatives so that they will understand and share her goals.

Where nurses implement change which affects their patients or clients and those who are involved with them, then they too must be part of the change process.

The change agents may become laggards too!

Example

A group of student nurses is discussing their experiences in a unit with the clinical nurse specialist. They have a number of complaints and weaknesses to bring out. The response of the senior nurse is to become defensive. 'You've no idea what it was like here years ago. I was brought in to make things better and we've made immense changes at great personal cost I can tell you! Of course, I don't expect you to appreciate all that, you don't remember how difficult it was in those days.'

The above example is the classic trap for the change agents. Resentment may occur when people still seem to want to change things. But, as was noted earlier, permanence is dead! The desire to change things will emerge continually, but at a cost to the change agent who may have accumulated so much power so as to become the conservative in the organisation.

There is a scene from a famous TV series of the 1960s and 70s, *Monty Python's Flying Circus* (1974), which mirrors this perfectly. Four 'old codgers' discuss their past, each trying to outdo the other in portraying how much hardship they endured, and how much easier the youngsters of today have it!

Without continuous education, moving on, new challenges, then those who have changed things may become complacent. The 'wallpaper effect' occurs; having visited a place so often, the blemishes and faults ceased to be noticed. Sometimes it takes a visitor to point them out. The trajectory of change has no terminus, only regular stops along the way to an infinite destination.

Financial implications

The process of change may exert financial pressures on the organisation, at the same time it may also save money. In times of economic stringency in health care, nurses are required more and more to put a good case forward if they wish to change things. If it is likely to save money, all well and good. The idea may be less well received if there is a higher cost implication. Sometimes changes which may make a demand for more money can be suppressed, and this is perhaps an understandable response by those who bear the responsibility of controlling the purse strings. However, the quality of life of staff and patients cannot be measured in terms of cost alone.

Sometimes costs can be met within existing resources, for example, by converting posts within a given staffing budget. In other settings, funds might be sought from external sources, such as charitable trusts. An example of this would be the well-known Oxford Nursing Development Unit's links with the Sainsbury Trust. However, examples of the latter type are rare, and even in the Oxford scheme there remained a heavy reliance upon the support of the staff in the organisation both to direct resources appropriately and to give the commitment. While Purdy and Wright (1988) have identified ways in which small units can set up nursing bursaries to identify external sources of cash, to generate income so that the limited resources of the organisation can be applied to the full, often, it is not the grand schemes which cause the biggest difficulties, but the day-to-day concern over payments to sustain the change process, for example:

supporting staff development, attendance at courses, conferences, etc.

providing equipment involved in the change, e.g., new nursing notes where a 'nursing process' approach is being developed

buying in teaching expertise from outside

use of staff time, either for teaching or development purposes, both teacher and taught will not be making their full contribution to the immediate service needs of the organisation

paying for resources to assist the learning/development process, e.g., providing books, journals, teaching equipment, as well as accommodation, furnishings, secretarial support and so on

The list of potential costs can be enormous. Sometimes it can be costed out fairly precisely – as in applications for research grants or development monies – while at other times the true cost can remain hidden or difficult to calculate.

However, where 'money' is a crucial factor, it seems that the following choices might need to be considered.

Can the change be managed within the existing resources?

Even if there is an initial cost, might the change eventually produce changes which may save money in the long term? (If so, how can this be demonstrated? Does the manager need a balance sheet of hard facts?)

What external sources of finance and support are available such as trust funds, research grants, bursaries? There are possibilities here worth exploring:

Check if the health authority itself has trust funds/bursaries available for assistance.

Contact the library or local authority for information on organisations willing to support innovations (e.g., the Guide to Company Giving (Directory of Social Change, 1986)).

Check local/national/nursing press for organisations offering assistance (e.g., the Nightingale Fund).

Investigate educational establishments for guidelines sources/for application for grants.

Contact appropriate professional bodies, institutes, health service organisations, etc., for avenues of funding.

Consider ways of raising funding locally, e.g., sponsorship schemes, fund-raising activities, getting support through the local press. Using networks of friends/local contacts who may be able to identify a possible sponsor.

These and more possibilities can be explored to support the costs of the change – much depends on the size of the scheme to be pursued, the length of time it will need, and the abilities of many individuals concerned with it to draw upon their entrepreneurial skills to raise money.

Case study II   Example of local bursary raising method

It was Mr Micawber in Dickens' *David Copperfield* who said: 'Annual income twenty pounds, annual expenditure nineteen ninety six, result happiness. Annual income twenty pounds, annual expenditure twenty pounds ought and six, result misery.' And many of the ideas we discussed in earlier articles cost money – lots of it.

The amount of money available for staff training is invariably limited, subject to severe restrictions, or absorbed for other use at times of crisis. In setting up a bursary, we had three essential principles in mind:

- The money would have to be generated from non-NHS sources
- It should be controlled by the nursing development unit (NDU) and not available to other hospital departments
- The policy for using the bursary, while being tight enough to include point two above, should also allow flexibility. A copy of the bursary guidelines appears at the end of the case study

The bursary committee meets monthly to monitor the accounts, the two nurse members having primary control over how money is spent. The cash is kept in a separate account from the health authorities, and earns interest. Final authorisation of payments is by the consultant nurse, with cheques being issued to the nurse concerned by the treasurer's office.

Currently we are seeking sponsorship for a large sum of money to fund some of our more adventurous projects. Meanwhile, we accrue funds from a wide variety of sources. It is our experience that people like to give money to a good cause, especially to nurses, and we have promoted this idea in the local community, telling people: 'This is *your* hospital, these are *your* nurses, help us to make better nurses.'

We also looked at the 'assets' we had which might attract investment. We had a new unit which attracted visitors eager to know how it was planned and managed; nurses wanted to know about our innovations – primary nursing, quality assurance, nursing process, nursing models and so on. So we asked: Did we have expertise which we could sell? It is true that in our hearts, we do not like behaving this way. Perhaps the traditional nurse in us feels that what we have should be freely shared with others. Unfortunately, while we may wish to give freely, events like courses and conferences cost money. We would like to think that a benevolent government would give us all the money we need to develop our staff, but this has not been the case in our nursing lifetime and we cannot imagine it being any different in the future.

We are also mindful of the danger that we might not get money from 'official' sources if we are generating income from elsewhere. We therefore make sure that we use existing budgets fully.

Profitable strategies were:

Fees for courses and conferences. We charge a reduced rate (usually half) to our own staff and ask more from outsiders. A recent afternoon seminar budget looked like this:

Speakers' fees and expenses	150
Providing drinks for staff	25
Expenditure	£175
Fees from local staff (£5 each, 40 participants)	200
Fees from nurses outside the H/A (£10 each, 40 nurses)	400
Gains	£600
	£600
	– £175
Profit	£425

While keeping costs to a minimum, and keeping fees as low as possible to attract people (who will often pay and attend in their own time), we were able to make a modest profit. We currently organise a one-day conference every three months, one or two seminars a month plus numerous workshops, and longer study sessions.

Donations from patients and relatives. Often money is offered to the wards, and the staff will ask how the donor wishes it to be used. Most relatives are happy to have part, if not all, their donation given to the bursary, which they see offering long-term benefit to staff and patients.

Sales of stationery and documentation. We copy these on site, and offer them for sale at a small profit to nurses who visit the unit or write and ask for them. They include the nursing process, nursing philosophy and guidelines on setting up an international exchange. Copies of our core care plans, for example, currently sell at £5 a full set (which includes more than 30 guidelines for use), and we have sold about 300 in the past year.

A fund raising committee. This organises all kinds of social events, sponsorships and so on. Profits from these are split 50/50, half going into the bursary and half going into trust funds to buy equipment.

Visitors' fees. We have special study days for visitors once a month, and these cover a variety of topics, including visits to the new unit and primary nursing. A fee is levied for these and an information pack given.

Donations. These come from local businesses, organisations, charitable organisations and drug firms. Some local factories have organised raffles or social events to raise funds for us.

Sponsorship. Two local pubs have 'adopted' the unit, and organise functions to raise money.

Consultancy fees. These are charged to companies that want to try out their products or conduct research on the unit although this is, naturally, carefully vetted and supervised. Some staff also teach in other health authorities or speak at conferences; the fees are added to unit funds when these activities occur during normal working hours.

The results we achieved were encouraging for the staff (we raised about £6 000 in the first six months), although we readily acknowledge that not all these activities are appropriate for every unit.

It is important to keep a close eye on expenditure. In general, we aim to keep more coming in than goes out. So far, the bulk of our costs have been on: course and conference fees to staff, everything from fees for degrees/diplomas to O-levels or one day conferences; supporting staff with the costs of the international exchange programme; buying equipment to assist the units' teaching programme (word processor, TV, video); subscriptions to journals; and buying books for the nursing development library.

We cannot rely on limited and declining NHS resources. Nurses have to become entrepreneurs and seek funds with which to help themselves. This is not a case of going out with a begging bowl, rather of adopting a more business-like approach and marketing what you have. It is not something we have gone into lightly, and it needs careful planning and management. For example, tying up all the loose ends regarding the bursary policy took about six months. However, it has paid off for us, and it is something well worth considering for those who despair of ever having enough money to support their staff.

The nursing development unit bursary
1 The general aim of the bursary will be to assist nurses with defraying the costs of their continued professional education.
2 The funds given to and arising from the bursary will be for the exclusive use of the professional development of nurses in Unit 1 nursing staff.
3 A fund will be established as an investment, the interest from which will release sufficient money annually to meet the needs of the bursary awards.
4 The bursary capital will be derived primarily from the work of the consultant nurse and the fund raising committee in creating links and sponsorship with the local community and industry and other income generating measures such as:
   • profits arising from conferences, courses and seminars

- visitor's fees and donations
- sale of copies of nursing documentation and research papers

5 Funding from the bursary will be open to all non-student nurses within the nursing development unit (care of the elderly).

6 The nurse seeking funds will set out details of the request in writing and submit it to the consultant nurse, in advance of the quarterly meetings, on or about the last day of March, June, September, December.

   a) The nature of the course of study/research project to be completed.

   b) The costs to be incurred.

   c) Details of any project work to be completed.

   d) The purpose of the course of study/research project.

7 The funds will be awarded after consideration by the bursary panel. Candidates may be requested to present themselves for interview before the panel if necessary.

8 The bursary panel's decision on the awarding of funds will be final.

9 The bursary panel will meet monthly to judge the worthiness of the project/course request submitted and may award funding in whole or in part to defray the costs.

10 The panel will consist of the consultant nurse, the clinical nursing officer, the unit's accountant and administrator as advisers. The function of this panel will be to agree upon who is to receive an award and how much money is to be made available.

11 The bursary panel will produce an annual report on projects and expenditure for the unit management team, which will include summaries of projects by candidates and the benefits gained.

12 The panel will monitor the level of the awards and the unit accountant will keep records of the accounts and available funds, and complete the appropriate procedures for the presentation of the cheque.

13 Candidates will be informed of the outcome of their applications within one month or after consideration at the first available panel meeting.

14 The awards will be made to defray the cost of items such as course fees, travel expenses, project typing, and other expenses as deemed appropriate by the panel. Funds to defray such costs maybe awarded in whole or in part at the discretion of the panel.

15 The Nursing Development Unit bursary will also be used to provide funds to purchase textbooks and pay for journal subscriptions for the NDU library. The sums to be released for such purposes will be agreed by the panel after request for relevant texts to be purchased have been submitted to them.

16 As sufficient funds become available, the bursary may also be used to support the cost of secretarial/research assistant for the NDU.

17 The bursary will also be used to underwrite the cost of conferences arranged on behalf of the NDU, although it is expected that all such conferences will be organised on a profit-making basis.

18 In the event of the failure to complete a course/research project, then any funds awarded will be required to be repaid to the NDU. The nurse will be required to sign an undertaking to this effect. Exceptions to this rule may be granted at the discretion of the panel after submission of relevant facts to them.

19 Any nurse accepting an award from the bursary must be prepared to:
    • provide a written summary of the course/project to the bursary awards committee on completion
    • submit details of the project to professional journals if considered suitable for publication
    • remain in employment of the Nursing Development Unit area for at least one year afterwards

20 The bursary is concerned solely with the award of funding; time off to attend the courses is not necessarily guaranteed, although applications will be viewed sympathetically. Request for study time must be made in the usual way through the appropriate clinical nursing officer.

21 Alterations to this bursary policy may be considered and approved with the agreement of the full panel.

22 Copies of this policy will be made available to all nursing settings in the Nursing Development Unit.

23 Advice and support on the submission of funding requests and the completion and writing up of projects will be provided by the consultant nurse.

The above case study gives an example of what can be achieved in one setting. Some elements of this, or all of them, might be helpful in supporting innovation in any setting.

Everything has its price, and changing nursing practice is no exception. Perhaps the most important aspect in this respect is the acceptance by the organisation as a whole, and those persons within it, that change is a continuous and acceptable normal part of its legitimate activities. When the culture of the organisation accepts change at this level, then the opportunity is so much greater for other parts of the change process to flow from it and through it.

When faced with the comment, 'We cannot afford to change', the riposte might well be, 'Can we afford not to?'.

References

Bailey, R. D. (1985). *Coping with Stress in Caring*. Blackwell Scientific Publications, Oxford.

Cherniss, C. (1980). *Staff Burnout: Job Stress in the Human Services*. Sage, London.

Cooper, C., Cooper R. and Eaten, L. (1988). *Living with Stress*. Penguin, Harmondsworth.

Department of Health and Social Security (1984–87). *The Health Service Ombudsman Reports*. DHSS, London.

Directory of Social Change (1986). *A Guide to Company Giving*. Bath Press, Bath.

Hardy, M. E. and Conway, M. E. (1978). *Role Theory: Perspectives for Health Professionals*. Appleton-Century-Croft, New York.

Lazarus, M. and Lannier, R. (1981). Stress related transactions between person and environment. *In* Dervin, L. A. and Lewis, M. (Eds), *Perspectives in Interpersonal Psychology*. Plenum, New York.

Martin, J. P. (1984). *Hospitals in Trouble*. Blackwell, Oxford.

Menzies, I. (1960). A case study on the functioning of social systems as a defence against anxiety. *Human Relations*, 13, 95–121.

Monty Python's Flying Circus (1974). *Four Yorkshiremen*. Monty Python Charisma Records, London.

Ottoway, R. N. (1976). A change strategy to complement new norms, new styles and new environment in the work organisation. *Personnel Review*, 5 (1), 13–18.

Purdy, E. and Wright, S. G. (1988). If I were a rich nurse. *Nursing Times*, 84(41), 36–8.

Salvage, J. (1985). *The Politics of Nursing*. Heinemann, London.

Salvage, J. (1988). *Facilitating Model-Based Nursing*. Paper given at Gateshead Nursing Models Conference. Unpublished.

Thomson, R. (1977). *The Psychology of Thinking*. Penguin, Harmondsworth.

Turrill, T. (1985). *Change and Innovation. A Challenge for the NHS*. Management Series 10. Institute of Health Service Management, London.

Wright, S. G. (1985). Change in nursing: the application of change theory to practice. *Nursing Practice*, 1 (2), 85–91.

6

Evaluation

'We seem to exist in a hazardous time,
Driftin' along here through space;
Nobody knows just how we began,
Or how far we've gone in the race.'

Ben King   *Evolution*

Evaluation

McFarlane and Castledine (1982) discuss the complex nature of nursing in its social and organisational setting and identify the problem of trying to define this human activity in simple terms. Given that the social and organisational role of the nurse is so diverse and complex, it follows that any attempt to evaluate the service provided, or any change in any part of it, will be problematic. This may be the reason why the concept of evaluation is so difficult for many nurses to understand and why the term is used to describe a wide range of activities from assessment to the carrying out of research methodologies.

Within the context of the nursing process, assessment is defined by McFarlane and Castledine (1982) as the identification of actual and potential patient problems on which the plan of care is based. Evaluation, as defined by these writers, is the process whereby actual patient outcomes are compared with the desired outcomes stated in the care plan. Thus, evaluation may be viewed as the collection and interpretation of information, by formal or informal means, to aid defensible decision making. It is also helpful to view evaluation as a continuum, with the making of value judgements at one end, and the rigorous methodologies of research at the other. In daily practice, the nurse may find him or herself at any point along this continuum in the evaluation of his or her own performance, the quality of care received by the patient, or the service offered by the institution.

Quantitative or qualitative methods: which do we choose?

Friend and Hayward (1986) and Lathleen *et al.* (1986) in their separate brief discussions on the evaluation of change in nursing outline two approaches. These approaches are categorised as: the quantitative or positivist model, and the qualitative or realist model. Like the change strategies discussed in Chapter 2, these approaches to evaluation are based on different and sometimes opposing assumptions.

The quantitative model is based on the assumption that scientific knowledge is obtainable only from data that can be directly experienced and verified between independent observers. Lathleen *et al.* (1986) argue that this approach is characterised by its commitment to an empirical base for scientific knowledge and to a notion of cause. The underlying assumptions of this approach is that its methods have a neutral value and that people can be studied as inert objects. The possibility that individuals and groups may initiate actions of their own accord, or in response to the complex interactions within groups, is overlooked in this model.

The purpose of the quantitative approach is to produce statements about causal relationships between discrete variables. This is achieved by isolating them from their natural surroundings and by artificially manipulating one or more of these variables. Statistical sampling is used to ensure that the cases studied reflect the population as a whole. This model has been widely used in the physical, biological and social sciences (Friend and Hayward, 1986; Lathleen *et al.*, 1986). It is the one most nurses will be familiar with through their basic and post basic education programmes and in their collaboration with medical colleagues' research programmes in clinical practice.

Quantitative methods are widely used in the current manpower planning programmes initiated by nurses throughout the country (Welsh Office, 1985). Examples of these include the ratings scales developed to determine patient dependency such as the Aberdeen system, the Naylor-Horne model for calculating the demand for and supply of nurses, the competency rating scales used to evaluate the process of nursing, and patient questionnaires distributed by the ward, unit or institution to determine patient satisfaction with the care received (All Wales Nurse Manpower Planning Committee, Welsh Office, 1985).

In contrast to the quantitative approach, qualitative methodologies focus on the subject's perceptions of the degree of change achieved that determines the success or failure of the innovation (Keyzer, 1985). Its methodologies tend towards internal rather than external evaluation. Parlett and Hamilton (1972) argued that to evaluate the changes brought about by innovations in complex human organisations the researcher has to leave his laboratory and study the group dynamics in the reality of the group's life. In this way, the qualitative approach acknowledges the emotional and social components of human behaviour ignored by the quantitative methods. By taking into account the effect individuals and organisational factors have on the behaviour of individuals and groups, the qualitative approach enables the evaluator to reinforce observation with discussion and background enquiry to promote an informed account of the innovation in action (Parlett and Hamilton 1972). This approach is still quite new to nursing research and evaluation, but examples of it do exist. Alexander (1983) used it to describe innovations in the organisation and delivery of the basic nurse education programme, Keyzer (1985) to describe the management of knowledge and change in the implementation of the nursing process, and Lathleen et al. (1986) to evaluate post-registration development schemes.

The question asked in the heading of this section was related to which of these approaches would most suit the evaluation of change. The answer to that question is both. In the reality of the work environment it is likely that both quantitative and qualitative methods will be used. There are no hard and fast rules to be applied and much will depend on what is to be evaluated and why it is being carried out. For example, if the organisation wants to know the numbers of nurses required to meet the patient's needs for care, it may use quantitative methods to calculate the demand for and supply of nurses, but semi-structured interviews, that is qualitative methods, to determine the patient's needs for care and satisfaction with the care received. It must also be remembered that in discussing the efficiency of change attention should also be drawn to the quality of the desired outcomes.

Performance indicators
One of the many changes currently taking place in nursing practice and education is the introduction of manpower planning and the evaluation of the way resources are managed by the nursing organisation. This move towards the planning of the demand for and supply of nurses and the identification of performance indicators by which the activities of institutions can be compared with each other dates back to the Platt Report (1964) on nursing education (HMSO, 1986). Then, as now, the emphasis on resource management stemmed from the problems of attracting new recruits, retaining qualified nurses and the public's changing demands on the National Health Service. Today, these factors have been reinforced by the stringencies of an economic recession. In their attempts to evaluate the efficiency and quality of their service, nurses must acknowledge the political, economic, organisational and professional factors which have determined the

role of the nurse in the hospital and community settings and the education programmes preparing them for these roles (Keyzer, 1985; White, 1985).

The term 'performance indicator' can be defined as a gauge or device for measuring an institution's and/or its component parts' level of success in achieving the objectives set for it in the organisation's strategic and operational plans. Performance indicators are tools which assist the nurse in her evaluation of the service offered to the public. Such an evaluation is orientated more towards the whole system rather than individuals who work in it. Appraisal of staff and the manner in which they utilise available resources are nevertheless part of the review of the whole system. Reid (1986) suggested that performance indicators could be considered as pointers that draw attention to many functions which include the use of resources and clinical activity, and cover the dimensions of economy, efficiency, accessibility and achievement of policy.

As with clinical practice, any attempt to monitor the service offered by the training institution must take into account the often divergent expectations held by the various groups who are charged with its organisation and delivery, and those who are consumers of the product. The issues and questions surrounding the standards these groups expect of the education service are central to the decisions taken in regard to the interpretation of the information gathered in the review of the service.

The who of evaluation

Identifying who is asking for the evaluation can help the nurse clarify where the demand for information is coming from and the nature of the data to be gathered. For example, when a doctor asks for an evaluation of the patient's progress, the data required are most likely to be concerned with the patient's response to medical intervention. If, however, a nurse asks for an evaluation of the same patient, the data required would reflect that patient's response to nursing interventions. For the nurse manager, the same patient's needs for care may be translated into information related to the number of nursing hours needed to provide care and, hence, the number of nurses needed to staff the clinical areas (Welsh Office, 1985). Thus different information about the same patient and his or her progress is required to meet the needs of the different groups providing input to the service offered. Identifying the source of the demand for information can determine what is to be evaluated, the method used to collect the data, and who is going to interpret the information provided.

An identification of the source of the demand for information can assist in describing the focus of the evaluation. Therefore, the 'who' of the evaluation can determine the object or subject of the process. For example, the teacher may focus attention on the student's ability to correlate theory to practice in the ward whereas the charge nurse may view the same student in terms of the skill mix required to meet the demands for care in the ward, and the nurse manager may look at the same student in terms of the cost of running the unit. In this way, the teacher would focus on the student's problem-solving skills, the charge nurse on his or her clinical expertise and place in the nursing team, and the manager on his or her salary in relation to the overall budget for the service. A different source can mean a different focus for the evaluation.

The source of the demand for the evaluation can also identify who will be making the judgement on the adequacy of the information gathered. This is of critical importance in that evaluation is about making value judgements on the worth of the service provided. The setting of goals for the National Health Service, the nursing service and its education programmes is a reflection of the values held by the various groups controlling and providing the service. In their every-day experience of the nursing service, patients, doctors, nurses, accountants, teachers and other groups make their subjective and objective evaluations of the service offered. Each of these groups evaluates the service from their own value systems and priorities for the service. Doctors have for a long time insisted on peer review, that is the quality of medical care evaluated from a medical perspective. That does not necessarily imply that what medicine accepts as a quality service will be accepted by the consumer of that service, or indeed by those who work with them.

Any evaluation of the nursing service and education programme based on the expectations of one group may be rejected by another. Thus an evaluation of the education programme by nurse teachers may be considered to be invalid by another organisational group whose value system differs from that of teachers. Kitson (1986) has argued that any evaluation of the quality of care provided by nurses should be viewed in the light of nursing values, that is, a nursing perspective. The same argument could also be made for an evaluation of the nursing education system. One of the problems in taking a nursing perspective is that nursing has for so long been dominated by the medical profession that little attention has been paid to nursing values by nurses. Previous reviews of the nursing service in research studies have been influenced by the nurse's need to approach the subject matter through the eyes of other disciplines, such as sociology. The current move towards the implementation of nursing models in practice and education, together with the greater access to higher education for nurses, should overcome this problem of agreement on what is and what is not a proper nursing perspective and the value placed on clinical practice and education by nurses.

It is also important to remember that values do not remain constant but change over time. What is held to be a quality service today may be rejected tomorrow. There are many examples of how nursing values have changed in recent times. Examples of the changes in nursing values are; the rejection of routinised care in favour of planned care, the demand for supernumerary status for learners, and a greater willingness to take the patient's perceptions of his needs for care into account. Whether or not the service provided by nurses meets the profession's expectations of the service depends greatly on the value it attaches to clinical practice and education. These professional values may be a reflection of the wider social values expressed by the population (Keyzer 1985). In defining the source of the evaluation, the nurse takes deliberate steps to describe the value system to be used in making decisions about the outcomes of the review and the acceptability of the information gathered.

Some of the difficulties of evaluation will now be illustrated by examining an extensive case study. The case study looks at some of the major factors in one setting where a change agent was employed to specifically alter an established care of the elderly setting.

Case study I

The conflict produced by the theory and practice gap in nursing appears to have detrimental effects upon both learners and teachers, and ultimately upon the care the patient receives (Birch, 1974; Bendall, 1975; Gott, 1984; Alexander, 1983).

One method to attempt to reduce this gap and its consequences is to create joint appointments 'to produce a job which encompasses both teaching and practice. The teaching often takes place in a separate setting, such as a School of Nursing or University, and the practice (which may also involve some 'clinical' teaching in a particular ward or in the community, where the post-holder takes direct responsibility for giving patient care)' (Wright, 1983).

Numerous accounts have now appeared documenting the development of joint appointments (Ashworth and Castledine, 1980; Walden, Sander and Gallant, 1982; Salvage, 1984; Wright, 1983; Balogh and Bond, 1984; Howden, 1985; Wenban, 1985). In one project (Wright, 1983; Wilkinson, 1983) the joint appointment role was developed specifically as a change agent, not only to affect nurse education, but also nursing practice. The 'Learning Climate' (Orton, 1981) on the care of the elderly unit could not be refashioned until the practice setting had been changed from an institutionalised approach to a patient-centred one. Thus it may be argued that in order to produce a learning climate (i.e., learner-centred environment) then the clinical setting must first and foremost be patient-centred. This would then match the ethos of the School of Nursing which tends to teach nursing as a patient-centred activity (Bendall, 1976). The job description for the joint appointments specifically incorporated these aims, and clearly designated the joint appointees as change agents, not only in producing an alternative educational model, but in changing practice as well. Items such as:

• 'Identify areas of concern related to nursing care and management of the ward which . . . affect the quality of care given, advise line managers of these areas and suggest possible solutions for discussion'.
• 'Develop a model of nursing based on the principle of individualised nursing care' (Wilkinson, 1983).

The setting originally chosen was a ward of 25 patients (male) dealing with acute medical problems of the over 65s. It was part of a unit of four wards and one day hospital (50 places) and came within the division of geriatrics. Significant changes took place in nursing practice. It is upon these changes that this study concentrates and in particular the methods by which they were achieved.

Change strategies

It is one thing to create a role with a specific brief of being a change agent – quite another to see the desired changes brought about. The choice of setting was quite deliberate, being a ward in an old workhouse building with facilities and an environment somewhat unsuited to the type of care being given. There was a heavy dependence on untrained nursing auxiliaries to meet staffing levels, and great difficulty in recruiting trained staff to the ward in particular and to the unit in general. There was an emphasis on task-centred care and a 'getting through the work' approach (Clark, 1978), producing a ritualised and institutionalised style of nursing. Coser (1963); Wells (1980); Miller and Gwynne (1972), for example, have illustrated the detrimental effect that such settings have upon patients and carers. In this instance, a specific change agent role (the joint appointment) was created to concurrently effect both care and learning.

It is possible to bring about change in people's behaviour by a direct authoritarian approach, i.e., by telling them how to do things differently. Rogers' (1969) influential philosophy, however, suggests that there are risks in this model. When the authority moves on, or becomes less effective, then there is a danger that a reversion to old norms and values takes place. Change can only become permanent if the desired values and attitudes have become a permanent part of the people in the care setting. One institutional framework can be broken down, but an alternative resilient framework must take its place if the changes are not to be swept away when the change agent departs.

For alternative goals and values to be reached – for people to come to a different view of their world – the egalitarian strategy is a neccessary tool. Kuhn (1970) sees knowledge as set in paradigms of ideas about the world. When a paradigm is in conflict with new knowledge it enters a state of crisis; a new way of looking at things is set up and a new paradigm established. An example of this would be the change in our concept of caring for and preventing pressure sores once our knowledge as to the cause of them had been developed.

Lewin's (1958) classic change theory defines 'no change' as a 'quasi-stationary equilibrium . . . a state comparable to that of a river which flows with a given velocity in a given direction during a certain time interval'. He describes social changes as comparable to a change in the velocity and the direction of that river, and sees the change process as having three basic steps:

- *Unfreezing* when the motivation to create some sort of change occurs, the impetus for this comes from three possible mechanisms:
- *lack of confirmation* or disconfirmation, i.e., the awareness of a need for change because expectations have not been met.
- *induction of guilt or anxiety*, i.e., uncomfortable feelings because of some action or lack of action.
- *psychological safety* when a former obstacle to change has been removed.
- *Moving* in which change is planned and initiated where cognitive re-definition occurs to look at the problem from a new perspective either through 'identification' or 'scanning' (the former solution provided by a knowledgeable peer; the latter solution found in a variety of sources).
- *Refreezing* in which change is integrated into the value system and stabilised into a new equilibrium.

In order to 'unfreeze' existing norms, and 'move' the staff to 'refreeze' into new norms, a tool to do the job is required. Many alternatives are available, and producing change in nursing is often a designated role for many practitioners, managers and educators. In this instance, however, a new role was created whose prime function was to change existing patterns of care and learning. In addition, a role emerged which straddled four diverse fields of nursing (practice, management, teaching, research) and which was financed and supported by two structures in nursing that are normally quite separately organised, namely the education and service sectors. The support and commitment of the managers in these sectors was to be a crucial factor in enabling the joint appointees to fully develop their role as change agents.

The idea of embodying change strategies in a specifically designated person – the change agent – is accepted by many authors on the subject (Rogers (1969) and Lewin (1958) among them). Ottoway's (1976) taxonomy (described in detail in this book) identifies a number of change agent types, and perhaps the joint appointees in this particular scheme had elements of all three, being change generators, implementors and adopters. However, as Salvage (1984) has noted, the experiment took place in a very ordinary setting. The posts were created out of existing budgets and existing staffing levels, with no special facilities or added benefits provided. Wilkinson (1984), as the Director of Nurse Education involved, has pointed out that she and the Director of Nursing Services deliberately took this approach. If similar changes were to be adopted elsewhere in the division, then resistance to change could be increased if the staff felt new behaviour was expected of them without the benefit of a perceived 'luxurious' setting.

In essence, the change strategy employed followed the work of Ottoway (1976) and Lewin (1958) closely. The change agents assisted in 'unfreezing' (Lewin 1958) established practices by working from the 'bottom up' (Ottoway 1976). A 'pilot site' was chosen (in this instance, one ward) to practice the new norms and style and with the joint appointees acting as onsite agents to introduce new skills and attitudes. Once the pilot site had rejected the old norms and reinforced the new, then it was ready to replicate itself within the organisation.

The individualised model of care arose eventually as a result of nurses coming together to look again at what they do; critically, sometimes cheerfully, sometimes uncomfortably. The 'coming together' may be deemed as an important feature, and much effort was needed to avoid the impression of an approach or change being imposed 'from above'. Ottoway's (1976) 'bottom up' approach requires nurses to feel they have rebuilt their own norms. The change agents (joint appointees) had to adopt a more subtle background role – dropping hints or a suggestion here, mentioning a reference or a piece of research there. There was also caution in the choice of words used, with an intention to avoid language which might seem academic or distant, to minimise the potential alienating effect. Written and verbal communication about nursing practice was deliberately couched in ordinary, everyday language. Staff meetings, sometimes as often as two or three times a week, were the main method of bringing all grades together, setting up a rich and fluid exchange of ideas.

The following is a summary of the change strategies.

- Staff meetings in the formal setting at work (all grades), day and night duty.
- Multidisciplinary meetings.
- Staff meetings (single grade).

- Informal staff meetings, social events out of work hours.
- Documentation of outcome of meetings, written agreement drawn up on philosophy, attitudes, practices.
- Change agents act as enablers, facilitators 'ideas men'.
- Language choice – simple, precise.
- Change 'atmosphere'; staff feel free to question, argue, debate.
- Tendency towards liberal/democratic management style, avoidance of autocracy.
- Progress reports, identification of patient/staff benefits, complimentary letters, etc., to reinforce change, encourage persistence.

The time factor needed to produce change has been mentioned, but it is worth noting that resistance to change may take much longer to overcome in some instances than in others. In settings where patient care is the end product of activity, how much time can be allowed for new norms of behaviour to be adopted? This is one instance where industrial models of change may conflict with social ones. Taking time for change may be permissible when the end product is an inert object, but what if the outcome involves human life? What if the undersirable activity is perhaps even dangerous to the patient? A variety of leadership styles are essential. While the liberal/democratic approach was emphasised, autocratic methods were sometimes necessary, especially in the early stages, to eradicate unsound practices. Thus while some issues could await the outcome of open debate and agreement, such as a reorganisation of the patient's day, others had to be resolved instantly through direct instruction, for example, the banning of routine application of Mercurochrome to pressure areas; even though this was backed up with some degree of discussion, and explanation was included.

As yet, little systematic evidence on the evaluation of joint appointments as change agents has become apparent, but from personal accounts (e.g., Ashworth and Castledine, 1980; Walden *et al.*, 1982; Wright, 1983; Balogh and Bond, 1984; Howden, 1985; Wenban, 1985), a general picture may be seen to emerge of factors which are important in supporting and enabling them to continue. A report by the King's Fund (1984) brought together many of these views in its meetings on joint appointees. Table 6.1 identifies the main sources of support to the change agents themselves and the prerequisite skills found necessary in this example:

- Possession of clinical, educational, managerial, research expertise (including awareness of change strategies) appropriate to the setting.
- Supportive, approachable education and service managers – tendency to informal relationships with them.
- Proven communication skills verbally/in writing.
- Physical and psychological stamina, patience.
- Clear philosophy of nursing and objectives.

- Peer group support of other change agents (e.g., King's Fund (1984) group).
- Knowledge of functioning of the health care system.
- Secretarial support.
- Positive personal/relationship supports in non-professional life.
- Clear sense of commitment to the job/perseverance.

Evaluation

Constant feedback also appears necessary between the change agents, the support managers, and the staff in the pilot site. It is of particular benefit if the staff can see an immediate result from their work. From the personal accounts mentioned above, it appears that enormous changes can accrue as the energies of staff are unleashed and redirected. A systematic evaluation of the effects of joint appointees as change agents has yet to emerge, but from the personal accounts a number of features appear to be common events in the pilot site over a period of time.

The points in Table 6.1 are, of course, very variable from setting to setting. In addition, the quality of nursing care is difficult to assess as so many variables are involved. For example, how far is patient turnover rate related to improvements/change in community support, medical practice, demographic changes and so on? However, a broad picture does seem to emerge when all the available information is brought together from those units where change agents have been active. They suggest a trend towards greater patient and staff involvement in care, the creation of more open care systems, and a general improvement in staff and patient satisfaction. It is perhaps not insignificant or mere coincidence that such a pattern develops in settings where change agents have been involved.

Other effects

Thus far it has been possible to draw upon the experience of one particular setting (Wright, 1983; 1984) where the strategies of Lewin (1958) and Ottoway (1976) have been employed, and to include settings where similar trends appear to have taken place. While the emphasis so far has been on changes in nursing practice, it appears from the above account that others are affected. Apart from student nurses, other staff too are drawn into a learning experience on wards which become both learner- and patient-centred. The support managers indicate that they too are affected (e.g., Shaw, 1984; Ashton, 1984) in developing alternative styles of management with the change agents. There appears to be a

Table 6.1 Reported effects in the pilot site.

Start $\longrightarrow$ Change $\longrightarrow$	After two years
Negative evaluations by learners	Positive learner evaluations
Patient turnover rate low/static with high readmission rate	Increased patient turnover, low readmission rate
High level of complaints from patients	Low level of patient complaints
High self-discharge rate by patients	Low self-discharge rates
Few complimentary letters on care	Increased compliment rate
Higher death/transfer rate	Reduced death rate, lower transfer rate to other (e.g., long-term) care
High staff turnover	Lower staff turnover
High staff sickness/absenteeism	Lower staff sickness/absenteeism
High staff work injury	Lower staff work injury
Higher patient accident rate	Lower patient accident rate
Incidence of pressure sores raised	Reduced pressure sore incidence
Incontinence levels high	Incontinence levels reduced
Absence of systematic care planning	Care planning organised
Ritualised/routine ward activity	Patient's day personalised
Task-centred nursing	Patient-centred nursing
Difficulty recruiting staff	Easier staff recruitment
	Increased staff job-satisfaction
	Increased student success in practical assessment
	Increased teaching input
Low level of patient and staff satisfaction	**Raised level of patient and staff satisfaction**

trend away from autocratic, authoritarian styles of management to more open, accessible and supportive methods.

The change agents themselves appear to adopt a more assertive style as nurses, expressing greater autonomy and advocacy in patient care, and it is as yet little explored how relationships of such nurses within the multidisciplinary team are defined. Certainly the potential for conflict, especially with the established medical order (Stein 1978), is very great when nurses indulge in the changing of practices and roles.

The change agents themselves appear to have a need for peer group support. In the case of joint appointees, the King's Fund (1984) suggests that they are in the business of 'role-creating' and therefore experience difficulties of feeling isolated, with no reference points to appeal to for guidance and support. In this instance, the desire to continue ways of enhancing help to each other has led to the formation of groups where mutual ideas and experiences can be shared (Wright, 1985; Thompson, 1985).

Finally, the pilot site becomes a source for change in other places – the wards of the nearby unit, often hospital wards, the division, and so on. It becomes a place where trained staff from other settings come for experiences to refresh their knowledge and return at some stage to their own places to act in turn as change

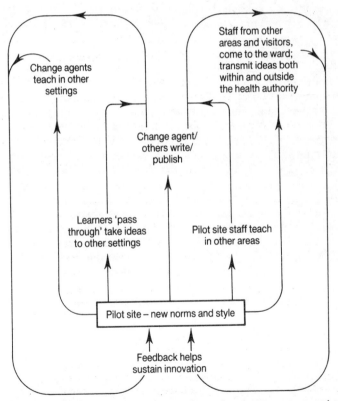

Fig. 6.1 Transmission of change from the change agent and the pilot site.

agents. This and other manifestations demonstrate clearly how Ottoway's (1976) concept of the pilot site emerges as the new norms and style are spread to other areas following the same principles. These new sites may not be exact replicas of the pilot site, but learn from and adapt their experience to their own place of work.

In addition, a feedback system is at work. Outside visitors attend the ward, and members of staff (especially the change agent) are involved in external teaching activities. This can lead to a continuous exchange of ideas, so that constant innovation is in evidence in the open system of the pilot site.

This case study has emphasised the role of a specifically created change agent. However, it needs to be stressed that the principles are applicable to many settings and many roles. As has been emphasised throughout this text, all nurses are change agents whether the term is specifically embodied in their job descriptions or not. The application of the theory and process of change in the hands of the skilled change agent appears to be a significant contributor to the production of new norms in the clinical setting (Pearson, 1985; Wright, 1986; MacGuire, 1988).

It is also important to note that a variety of criteria had to be selected to evaluate the outcome, often profoundly affected by the nurse's own value systems (e.g., the assumption that introducing 'care planning' is a good thing). However, by identifying factors *pertinent to a particular setting* (e.g., looking at patient admission/discharge rates may not be relevant) and gathering data on these before, during and after the change process, an evaluation of the change process can be conducted. Rarely will *one* factor provide adequate evaluation, depending on how much is to be changed. In general, the broader the objectives being set, the more the scope for gathering in data for evaluation.

Factors in the setting can be examined for evaluation purposes, but so too can elements in the job description and in performance indicators. A recent ENB (1987) package has examined change theory in depth and gives suggestions on looking at not only the outcomes of change, but also evaluation of the change process itself to see if the methods shown were developed correctly.

Anatomy of an innovation
A series of points to consider to analyse whether change was successful or not (after ENB, 1987).

1 Assess the attributes of the innovation you are recalling, in terms of:
   a) relative advantage
   b) compatibility
   c) communicability
   d) simplicity
   e) trialability
   f) observability
   g) relevance
   Did your innovation fail on one, or several, of these counts? Looking back, could the innovation have been better conceived?

2 Assess the 'ripeness for change' of the environment into which you attempted to introduce the change. Did it show:
   a) openness?
   b) interpersonal and informational linkages?
   c) freedom from organisational constraints?
   d) supportive leadership?
   e) trust?
   If your innovation failed on one or more of these counts, there may be problems in the environment that will hinder future attempts at innovation. If you suspect this to be the case, you may find that it helps to make a more general review of organisational health. Any barriers to change, personal or organisational, that you can note will be relevant to the review.

3 Assess the 'users' of the innovation in terms of their readiness to change. What proportion (or who) are:
   • innovators?
   • early adopters?
   • early majority?
   • later majority?
   • laggards?
   • rejecters?
   To what extent do you think users' readiness to adopt the innovation was affected by:
   a) their sense of ownership (or lack of it) of the change?

  b) their informal personal contacts (or lack of them) over the change?

  c) the involvement (or lack of it) of opinion leaders?

  d) the information and support (or lack of it) that they received in connection with the change?

4 Assess the change strategy used. Would you describe it as:

  a) rational–empirical?

  b) power–coercive?

  c) normative–re-educative?

  d) a combination?

Did you use different strategies over a period if the first one failed?

5 Assess the success of the change agent(s) involved in the innovation. How well did they carry out their functions of:

- diagnosing the problem?
- identifying and clarifying goals?
- developing appropriate strategies and tactics?
- developing good working relationships with users?

How many of the characteristics of a successful change agent did they possess?

- effort
- client orientation
- compatibility
- empathy
- use of opinion leaders
- credibility
- effort with regard to evaluation
- experience
- reflectiveness
- self-awareness
- supportiveness

It is important, therefore, to look at change not only from the perspective of its observable results, but also at 'the living, breathing people who experience it' Toffler (1973).

References

Alexander, M. F. (1983). *Learning to Nurse*. Churchill Livingstone, Edinburgh.
Ashton, S. (1984). Managing at a distance. *Senior Nurse*,1(31), 22–4.
Ashworth, P. and Castledine, G. (1980). Joint service–education appointment in nursing. *Medical Teacher*, 2(6), 295–9.
Balogh, R. and Bonds, S. (1984). An analytical study of a joint clinical teaching service appointment on hospital ward. *International Journal of Nursing Studies*, 21(2), 81–99.
Bendall, E. (1975). *So you passed, Nurse*. Royal College of Nursing, London.
Bendall, E. (1976). Learning for reality. *Journal of Advanced Nursing*, 1(1), 3–9.
Birch, J. (1974). *To Nurse or not to Nurse*. Royal College of Nursing, London.
Clark, M. (1978). Getting through the work. *In* Dingwall, R. and McIntosh, J. (Eds), *Readings in the Sociology of Nursing*. Churchill Livingstone, Edinburgh.
Coser, R. L. (1963). Allienation and the social structure. *In* Tucker, D. and Kaufert, J. (Eds), *Readings in Medical Sociology*. Tavistock, London.
English National Board (1987). *Managing Change in Nursing Education: Pack One: Preparing for Change*. ENB, London.
Friend, P. and Hayward, J. (1986). *Report of the Nursing Process Evaluation Group*. NERU Report No. 5. King's College, London.
Gott, M. (1984). *Learning Nursing*. Royal College of Nursing, London.
Her Majesty's Stationery Office (1986). *The Platt Report* (1964). HMSO, London.
Howden, C. (1985). Community links. *Senior Nurse*, 2(8), 6–8.
Keyzer, D. M. (1985). *Learning Contracts; The Trained Nurse and the Implementation of the Nursing Process*. Phd Thesis, London University.
King's Fund (1984). *Joint Clinical Teaching Appointments in Nursing*. Project paper No. 52. King's Fund Centre, London.
Kitson, A. L. (1986). Indicators of quality in nursing care – an alternative approach. *Journal of Advanced Nursing*, 11, 133–44
Kuhn, T. (1970). The structure of scientific resolution. *International Encyclopaedia of Unified Science*, 2 (2).
Lathleen, J., Bradley, S. and Smith, G. (1986). *Professional Development Schemes for Newly Registered Nurses*. NERU Report No. 4. King's College, London.
Lewin, K. (1958). The group decision and social change. *In* Maccoby, E. (Ed). *Readings in Social Psychology*. Holt, Rinehart and Winston, London.
MacGuire, J. M. (1988). I'm your nurse, here's my card. *Nursing Times*, 84 (30), 32–6.
McFarlane, J. K., Castledine, G. (1982). *A Guide to the Practice of Nursing using the Nursing Process*. The C. V. Mosby Co., St Louis.
Miller, E. J., Gwynne, G. V. (1972). *A Life Apart*. Tavistock, London.
Orton, H. (1981). *The Ward Learning Climate*. Royal College of Nursing, London.

Ottoway, R. M. (1976). A change strategy to implement new norms, new style and new environment in the work organisation. *Personnel Review*, 5(1).

Parlett, M. and Hamilton, D. (1972). *Evaluation as Illumination: A New Approach to the Study of Innovatory Programmes*. Occasional Paper. Centre for Research in the Education Sciences, University of Edinburgh.

Pearson, A. (1985). *The Effects of Introducing New Norms in a Nursing Unit; An Analysis of the Process of Change*. Unpublished PhD Thesis, University of London.

Reid, E. (1986). Performance indicators. *Nursing Times*, 82(37), 44–8.

Rogers, C. (1969). *Freedom to Learn*. Merrill, Columbus, Ohio.

Salvage, J. (1984). An experiment in co-operation. *Senior Nurse*, 1(7), 14–16.

Shaw, H. (1984). Practising what you preach. *Senior Nurse*, 1(23), 22–3.

Stein, L. (1978). The doctor-nurse game. *In* Dingwall, R. MacIntoch. J, (Eds), *Readings in the Sociology of Nursing*. Churchill Livingstone, Edinburgh.

Thompson, G. (1985). Society for nurses on advanced practice – a report. *Nursing Practice*, 1(1), 63–4

Toffler, A. (1973). *Future Shock*. Pan Books, London.

Walden, E. Sander, R. and Gallant, K. (1982). Sharing the pleasure and the pain. *Nursing Times*, 78 (21), 833–6.

Wells, T. (1980). *Problems in Geriatric Nursing*. Churchill Livingstone, Edinburgh.

Welsh Office (1985). *The First Report of the All Wales Nurse Manpower Planning Committee*. WHC, 85/32.

Wenban, P. (1985). One school of thought. *Senior Nurse*, 2(8), 8–9.

White, R. (Ed.) (1985). *Practical Issues in Nursing, Past and Present and Future*, Vol. 1. John Wiley and Sons, Chichester.

Wilkinson, K. E. M. W. (1983). A blueprint for a joint appointment. *Nursing Times*, 79(42), 29–30.

Wilkinson, K. E. M. W. (1984). The work in question. *Senior Nurse*, 1(28), 17–20.

Wright, S. G. (1983). The best of both worlds. *Nursing Times*, 79(42), 25–9.

Wright, S. G. (1984). Quality matters. *Senior Nurse*, 1(9), 16–19.

Wright, S. G. (1985). Comment. *Nursing Standard*, 7 February.

Wright, S. G. (1986). *Building and Using a Model of Nursing*. Edward Arnold, London.

Conclusion: Nurses and the power to change

'O! It is excellent
To have a giant's strength, but it is tyrannous
To use it like a giant.'

Shakespeare *Measure for Measure*

To effect change it has so far been argued that nurses need both the knowledge and resources to do it. By virture of sheer numbers, nurses could represent a gigantic force for social change. Even given the knowledge, would nurses *en masse* still use it? A recent ENB (1987) text asks, 'How effective is nursing in developing and deploying the necessary skills to take control over its own destiny? Do sufficient numbers of nurses know how 'the system' ticks, what 'power' is and how to use it, and how to function as change agents?'.

Knowledge of change would not only equip nurses to be better change agents, it would also help them (knowing why, how and where it is coming from) to resist change when appropriate. Resistance to change is not always a negative process, even if it might annoy those seeking to change things, because it 'fires the proponents of change to justify and promote the reasons for their proposals' (ENB, 1987). After all, change is not always for the better, and resistance is sometimes well-founded, given the pitfalls in nursing history.

Teaching nurses how to be change agents rarely finds its way into the curriculum of schools of nursing. True, some argument might, with some justification, be put forward that there is little time to squeeze it in among other, apparently more pressing, needs. However, might there not also be some reluctance on the part of those in power to include this subject? The established system of health care, might at the very least, be rocked to its foundations. There are 500 000 nurses in the UK – just imagine the effect, not only on nursing in the health service, but in society as a whole, if such a vast army of skilled change agents was unleashed upon them!

Meanwhile, nursing is held in check. As a female dominated occupation, it is inhibited in its potential in a society which still largely functions and sets priorities around male values. The discipline is still affected by the pervasive (male) medical model which prefers to keep nurses in their place (Salvage, 1985). The future of nursing is inextricably linked with the assertive role of the woman. Change in nursing is coming painfully slowly in a system which still adheres to hierarchical, bureaucratic values espousing obedience, routine and authority.

To move away from this is not to advocate anarchy, but to wean nursing away from the 'narcissistic mirror offered by medicine' (Oakley, 1984) so that it occupies its rightful place in the chorus of health care. Moving nursing into a position where it would dominate all other professions would be as unhelpful to those it serves – the patients or client – as is nursing's currently oppressed status. Professional power tends to corrupt into a 'conspiracy against the laity' (Freidson, 1970). The professional power to change things, which this book has espoused, seeks not mastery but partnership; with clients and other disciplines. In this sense, nursing cannot, and must not, adhere to the traditional sociological definition of a profession. If nursing does this, it will become like the pigs in *Animal Farm* (Orwell, 1951), 'Twelve voices were shouting in anger, and they were all alike. No question, now, what had happened to the faces of the pigs. The creatures outside looked from pig to man, and from man to pig, and from pig to man again; but already it was impossible to say which was which'.

At the same time, seeing nursing as in conflict – with management, other professions, and with clients – is an outmoded paradigm. It is helpful to no one to see the position of nurses simply as the result of dominance by others. The picture is far more complex, far more subtle. Nursing, after all, is still quite young, as professions go, with enormous potential for the future.

At this stage, it would be useful to reconsider some of the salient points as to the ways in which nurses can become effective change agents.

• Acquire knowledge. Attend a course or conference, read widely, take out a learning contract with a teacher or mentor, start work on a distance learning package, learn about change theory. Get to know more about how you and the organisation ticks. Take a course in self-awareness and assertiveness. Awareness of your own situation is the first step on the road to changing the world around you (Freire, 1973). Learn who the key people are in your organisation and how to lobby them for support.

• Own the process of change. Work with colleagues in small or large groups. Set up a quality circle (Christie, 1986), for example, to determine for yourself the things you would like to change. Set out your goals and map out how you wish to achieve them.

• Learn about, select and use a change strategy. What is the best position to be in to effect change? What can you do where you are now? Assess, plan, implement and evaluate.

• Look after yourself. Check that what you wish to do lies within the framework of your accountability. Take time for yourself. Nothing is so important that it burns you out, drains you completely, or destroys your valued relationships.

• Give it time. Changing the organisation of even one ward or one small unit can take years. Don't be disappointed if it isn't all perfect overnight.

• Form a conspiracy. Get colleagues, managers, teachers, on your side. Work slowly, deliberately through the power of the group to achieve your goals. Act at both a personal and political level.

• Accept that change is evolutionary; be prepared for hold-ups, set-backs. Be flexible, prepared to adapt your strategy, think again, change course.

• Don't feel guilty if it doesn't all go right. It isn't all your fault. Look back upon what you have done well, value it, cherish it, and do this on a regular basis so the progress you have made, however small, is not lost sight of. There may be mountains ahead, but many hills lie behind that you have already climbed.

• Set your sights within your range. Aim for things which you know you *can* do. Start small and work up to the big goals, achieving each step as you go and avoiding disappointment.

• Check up on your own skills. Becoming a change agent is a lifelong process. Engage others as you go along. Develop your communication skills. Give praise to colleagues rather than criticism.

• Don't underestimate the qualities you need to change things. Combine you own drive with physical and psychological stamina. Keeping yourself physically fit is often as important as looking after your personal and professional relationships.

• Keep up to date and help colleagues to do the same. Disseminate your ideas using your colleagues. Provide books, journals, written information, so that those involved in the change process can become as enlightened as you are!

- Focus on one place at a time. Set up a pilot site and use it as the base to achieve your aims. This can itself become a transmission site for new ideas (see Chapter 6).

- Plan an evaluation strategy for before, during, and after the change process. This will help justify your case, and can give you and your colleagues the evidence for achievement.

- Document what you do. Write about it and let others know about it. Consider it for publication, others can learn from your experience.

- Become political, both with a big and small 'p'. It is not only important to influence your own organisation but to influence others in power too. Next time the politicians call, ask them what they propose to do about *your* difficulties. If nurses become 'involved in and participate in political decision-making through the nursing organisations and in the political parties, I believe they will be an unstoppable force for change' (Clay, 1987).

- Map out your own career. Seek careers advice. Get yourself into a position of power best suited to effect the kind of changes you want.

- Explore your values, clarify your ideals; they are a real source of strength in difficult times.

To be a change agent is a difficult task, but it provides a path full of challenge, opportunities and possibilities – they are the things which make us human. As a change agent, the nurse has to draw upon all the resources of physical and psychological stamina; this may test your credibility to its limits, along with your powers of intellect and communication. Subtlety, guile, imagination, empathy, resourcefulness: these are the tools, the stock in trade of those who would change things, creating a climate of change not only among small groups of colleagues, but ultimately to a change culture that exists at all levels of the organisation. Often the organisation is strong and repressive, but at other times it is ripe for change as, for example, when new government policies destabilise existing systems and provide an expectation of change. Nurses have to be ready to move in when the ideal opportunity arrives – when they do not, others are only too ready and willing to fill the vacuum.

There are many possible methods of attempting change in nursing. With its hierarchical system of organisation, its immense size in terms of numbers, and its place in the establishment under the umbrella of health care, it is perhaps one of the most difficult areas to innovate, especially where established attitudes and practices are challenged. Yet it is precisely these reasons which can contribute to nursing strength in the potential for change.

It may be argued that success, where it is achieved, is due in no small measure to those change agents with the courage and energy to commit themselves to it, and to those who support them. This book has attempted to explore ways of implementing change in a planned and systematic way, and with a sound theoretical base. Combined with the personal and intuitive powers of each nurse, change is a powerful force. It is contended that, although the style and emphasis of the change method may differ, change must be organised in this way if it is to attain its goal of infusing new norms and practices into the system. Unplanned and disordered change may lead to dissipation and wastage of much energy at great personal cost. The price of change where this occurs may be considered unacceptable. When nurses take on their role as change agents, then change in nursing practice is achievable. In this way, innovative, creative and personalised nursing can emerge when those features which are changed become an accepted part of the new order. We owe it to ourselves. We owe it to our patients. Nurses can do it.

References

Christie, H. (1986). Quality circles – staff ideas are your richest resource. *Health Service Options*, pp. 17.

Clay, T. (1987). *Nurses, Power and Politics*. Heinemann, London.

English National Board (1987). *Managing Change in Nursing Education Pack One: Preparing for Change*. ENB, London.

Freidson, E. (1970). *The Profession of Medicine*. Dodd-Mead, New York.

Freire, P. (1973). *Education: The Practice of Freedom*. Writers and Readers Publishing Cooperative, London.

Oakley, A. (1984). The importance of being a nurse. *Nursing Times*, 12, 24–6.

Orwell, G. (1951). *Animal Farm*. Penguin, Harmondsworth.

Salvage, J. (1985). *The Politics of Nursing*. Heinemann, London.

Index